Minimally Invasive Spine Surgery - Advances and Innovations

Edited by Mick Perez-Cruet

Published in London, United Kingdom

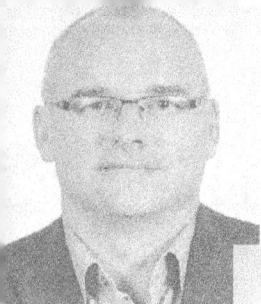
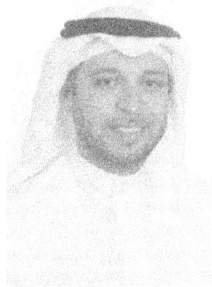
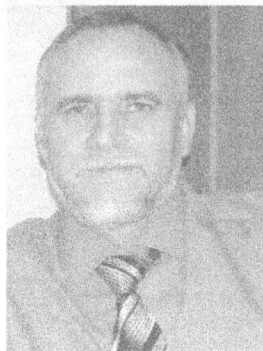
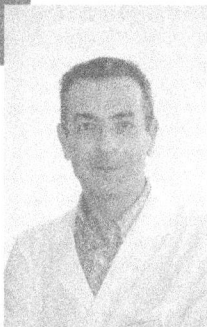
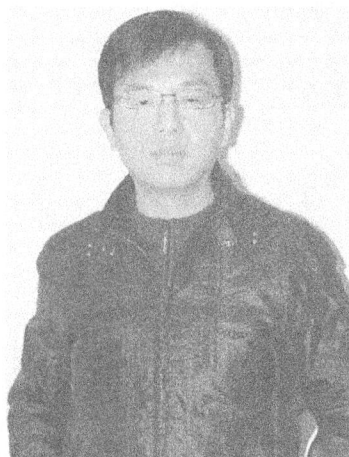
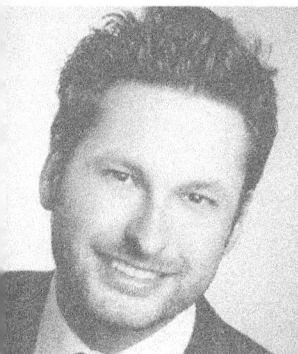
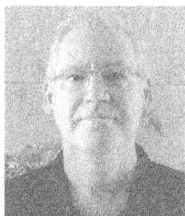

IntechOpen

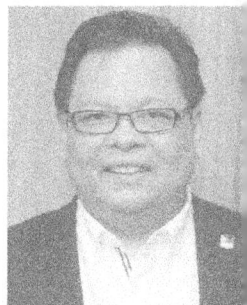
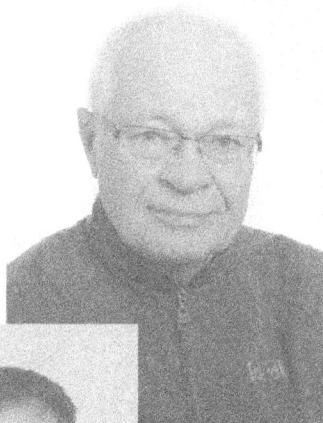
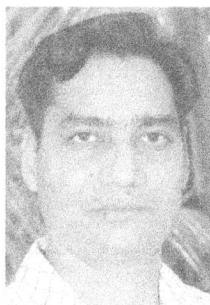
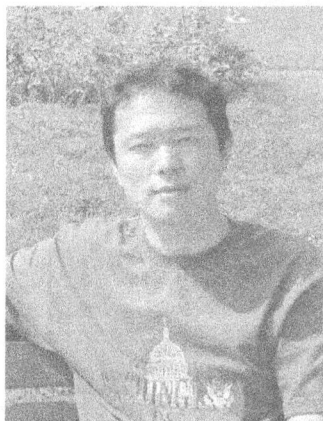
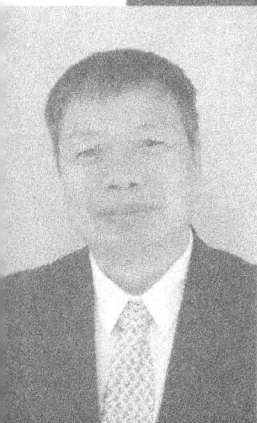
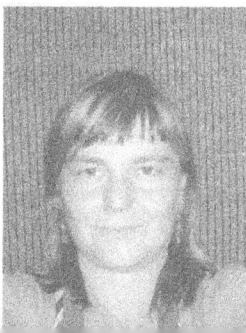

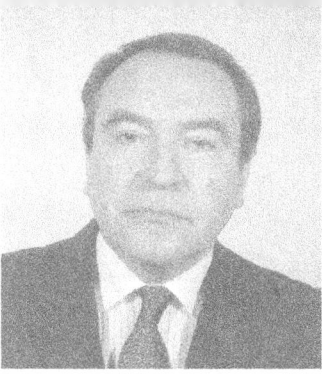

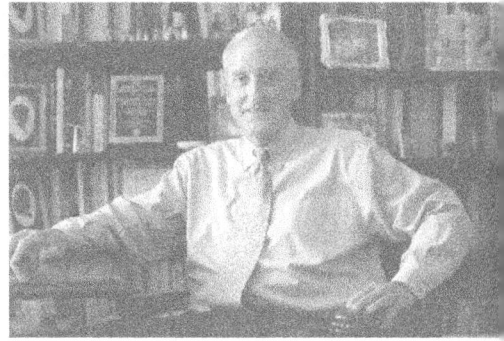

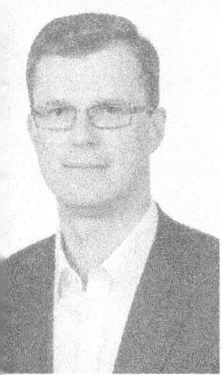

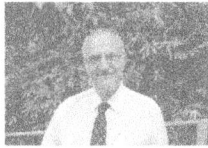

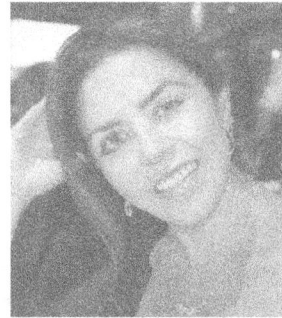

Supporting open minds since 2005

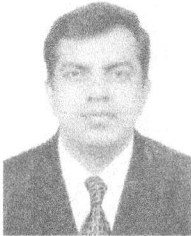

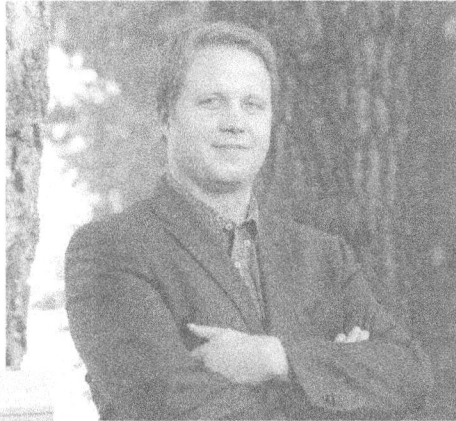

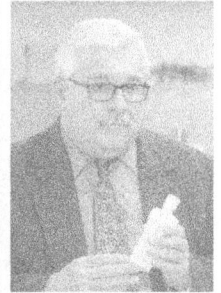

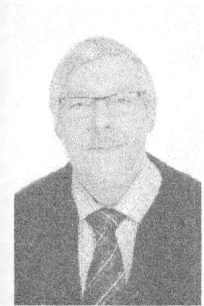

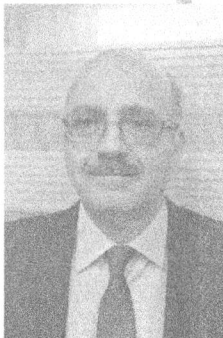

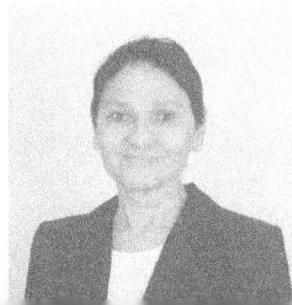

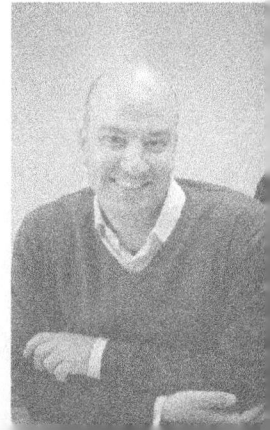

Minimally Invasive Spine Surgery - Advances and Innovations
http://dx.doi.org/10.5772/intechopen.93743
Edited by Mick Perez-Cruet

Contributors
Donald Blaskiewicz, Luis D. Diaz-Aguilar, Ronald Sahyouni, Pablo Pazmiño, Kee Kim, Amir Goodarzi, Tejas Karnati, Edwin Kulubya, Daniel J. Denis, Edna E. Gouveia, Mansour Mathkour, Erin McCormack, Jonathan Riffle, Olawale A. Sulaiman, Siavash Beiranvand, Farshad Hasanzadeh-Kiabi, Daniel K. Fahim, Eric R. Mong, Sheeraz A. Qureshi, Ram Kiran Alluri, Ahilan Sivaganesan, Avani S. Vaishnav, Richard N.W. Wohns, Mick Perez-Cruet, Ramiro Pérez de la Torre, Siddharth Ramanathan, Jason M. M. Highsmith

Notice
Statements and opinions expressed in the chapters are these of the individual contributors and not necessarily those of the editors or publisher. No responsibility is accepted for the accuracy of information contained in the published chapters. The publisher assumes no responsibility for any damage or injury to persons or property arising out of the use of any materials, instructions, methods or ideas contained in the book.

First published in London, United Kingdom, 2022 by IntechOpen
IntechOpen is the global imprint of INTECHOPEN LIMITED, registered in England and Wales, registration number: 11086078, 5 Princes Gate Court, London, SW7 2QJ, United Kingdom
Printed in Croatia

British Library Cataloguing-in-Publication Data
A catalogue record for this book is available from the British Library

Additional hard and PDF copies can be obtained from orders@intechopen.com

Minimally Invasive Spine Surgery - Advances and Innovations
Edited by Mick Perez-Cruet
p. cm.
Print ISBN 978-1-83962-301-1
Online ISBN 978-1-83962-302-8
eBook (PDF) ISBN 978-1-83962-303-5

We are IntechOpen,
the world's leading publisher of
Open Access books
Built by scientists, for scientists

6,000+
Open access books available

146,000+
International authors and editors

185M+
Downloads

Our authors are among the

156
Countries delivered to

Top 1%
most cited scientists

12.2%
Contributors from top 500 universities

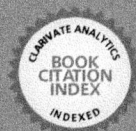

Interested in publishing with us?
Contact book.department@intechopen.com

Numbers displayed above are based on latest data collected.
For more information visit www.intechopen.com

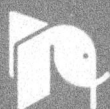

Meet the editor

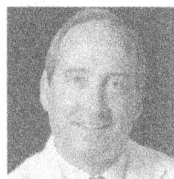

Dr. Mick Perez-Cruet is an internationally recognized pioneer in the treatment of spinal disorders using minimally invasive surgical techniques. His experience spans more than thirty years. He is vice chairman and professor of the Department of Neurosurgery, Oakland University William Beaumont School of Medicine, MI. He is one of the core faculty for the recently established ACGME Neurosurgery Residency Program at the same university. He is the Beaumont Neurosurgeon Champion for the Michigan Spine Surgery Improvement Collaborative (MSSIC), which is the largest comprehensive spine surgery outcome registry in the country. He dedicates much of his time to teaching neurosurgeons, fellows, residents, and medical students. He has served as the Michigan delegate to the Council of State Neurosurgical Societies (CSNS) for more than twenty years, was president of the Michigan Association of Neurological Surgeons (MANS), and holds several administrative positions within Beaumont. Additionally, he is president and founder of the Minimally Invasive Neurosurgical Society (MINS), a nationally recognized organization that promotes improved patient outcomes through surgeon teaching, cadaveric labs, and research to promote minimally invasive spine and cranial procedures.

Contents

Preface

Advances in minimally invasive spine surgery (MIS) have improved patient outcomes for a variety of pathologies affecting the spinal column. These advances all have the same goal, which is to improve patient outcomes by reducing approach-related morbidity. Patients can have quicker recoveries and return to normal active lifestyles by preserving the normal anatomical structures and or motion of the spine when performing spine surgery. These goals are increasingly becoming the required objectives of patients when seeking out surgeons to perform their spine procedures. Those surgeons who know how to treat patients in a minimally invasive fashion will grow their practices and help many suffering patients effectively. There has been a boom in MIS treatments and advancements in this area have accelerated rapidly. This book teaches physicians how to treat patients using MIS, improve outcomes, and quickly return patients to full and active lifestyles.

In this book, we list some of the latest advancements and developments in MIS. This is by no means a complete textbook on MIS and additional materials are needed to keep up with this rapidly advancing field.

The first section begins with chapters on cervical approaches, including outpatient cervical arthroplasty as well as novel arthroplasty devices that mimic the true motion of the human cervical spine. These newer technologies allow for motion in all six planes including flexion, extension, lateral rotation, and compression. The intervertebral disc is not a ball and socket joint like the hip or knee; therefore, for arthroplasty devices to truly work, compression and limited motion as seen in the anatomical annulus fibrosis and nucleus pulposus of the intervertebral disc should be reproduced in an arthroplasty device.

In the second section, chapters discuss minimally invasive and novel approaches for treating the pathology of the thoracic spine.

In the third section, chapters address minimally invasive lumbar approaches. This is the largest section since most surgical pathology we treat is in the lumbar spine. It discusses novel minimally invasive approaches that treat very common spinal conditions like lumbar stenosis and spondylolisthesis. These approaches preserve the normal anatomy of the lumbar spine, including the spinous processes and the paraspinal muscle attachments to the spinous process and lamina. This is critical in preventing stresses on adjacent levels, which can lead to joint and ligamentum flavum hypertrophy requiring additional and costly reoperations. Patients clearly recover faster and return to active lifestyles with these procedures that preserve much of the normal anatomy and function of the lumbar spine. Though we still do not entirely understand the underlying physiological etiology of spinal stenosis, fusing the segment while preserving much of the normal anatomy of the spine, as is explained in this book, can lead to long-lasting, excellent outcomes for these patients. This includes those patients suffering from multi-segmental spinal stenosis. The traditional procedures where the spinous process is removed over multiple segments can lead to high rates of adjacent segment disease, scarring, and failed laminectomy syndrome. This can result in considerable patient suffering and poor outcomes. If the content of this book can help these patients alone, then it has achieved a major goal in advancing the spine field.

The fourth section includes one chapter on treating spinal malignancy in a minimally invasive fashion. This chapter not only explores novel approaches but also focuses on treatment that can help to reduce morbidity while improving survival and outcomes for patients suffering from spinal malignancy.

The final section on minimally invasive assisted robotic spine surgery (MARSS) is a rapidly growing area in MIS. Using robots, spinal instrumentation can be applied accurately and precisely while preserving the normal anatomical structures of the spine. Indeed, more recent technology is advanced to the point where the surgeon can literally peer through the spine as if having x-ray vision. The result is that there is no longer a need to strip away and destroy critical anatomical structures of the spine like muscles, ligaments, bones, and joints to view the bony anatomy. These structures are critical to the long-term health of the spine and preserving their form and function can greatly improve patient outcomes, reduce the need for reperforming spine surgery, and quickly returns patients to their full and active lifestyles, which is the ultimate goal.

Mick Perez-Cruet, MD, MS
Vice Chairman and Professor,
Director, Minimally Invasive Spine and Spine Program,
Department of Neurosurgery,
Oakland University William Beaumont,
School of Medicine,
Auburn Hills, Michigan

Department of Neurosurgery,
Michigan Head and Spine Institute,
Southfield, Michigan, USA

Section 1

Minimally Invasive Cervical Approaches

Cervicogenic Headache Hypothesis and Anterior Cervical Decompression as a Treatment Paradigm

Amir Goodarzi, Edwin Kulubya, Tejas Karnati and Kee Kim

Abstract

Cervicogenic headaches are a controversial clinical entity that affect many patients suffering from cervical spondylosis. Understanding the pathogenesis and identifying the nociceptive sources of cervicogenic headaches is critical to properly treat these headaches. A multimodal approach is necessary to treat these headaches using a variety of medical tools. Surgical interventions are reserved for patients that fail maximal medical therapy. The anterior cervical spine surgery has shown promise in the treatment of cervicogenic headaches and this success has hinted at a ventral source of nociceptive pathology. Continued research and development are required to improve outcomes in patients suffering from cervicogenic headaches.

Keywords: cervicogenic, headache, sinovertebral nerve, neck pain, referred pain

1. Introduction

Cervicogenic headaches (CGH) were first recognized as a distinct pathologic entity in the 1980's to describe a group of patients suffering from headaches that occurred in the presence of cervical spondylosis and neck pain. The diagnostic criteria and pathogenesis of CGH have remained contentious with many competing hypotheses described in recent years. However, despite the knowledge gap and lack of a comprehensive understanding of the underlying pathogenesis, significant clinical evidence has been published on successful treatment paradigms for CGH. Clinicians have used a variety of approaches in treating cervicogenic headaches including both medical and surgical techniques. Anterior cervical decompressive surgery is a minimally invasive procedure that has demonstrated promising and durable results for symptom relief in CGH. In this chapter we review the pathogenesis, diagnosis, and some of the minimally invasive surgical techniques used to treat cervicogenic headaches.

2. Current understanding of cervicogenic headache pathogenesis

The term cervicogenic headache (CGH) was first conceived in 1983 by Sjaastad et al. to describe patients experiencing episodic headaches that were triggered by stereotypical neck movements in the setting of cervical pathology (e.g. radiculopathy, myelopathy, soft tissue lesions) [1]. Sjaasted et al. observed that these headaches were accompanied by neck pain, neck rigidity, and dysautonomia. The dysautonomic symptoms included unilateral lacrimation, rhinorrhea, tinnitus, blurred vision, flushing of the face, photophobia, phonophobia, nausea, and vomiting [1, 2]. Most peculiarly, many patients noted myofascial trigger points in the neck, ipsilateral to the headaches, that could precipitate their symptoms with great intensity [1–3].

Over the last decade, there has been continued controversy regarding a consistent definition for CGH. However, a common framework has recently been established by the International Headache Society's Headache classification (ICHD-3). The ICHD-3 defines CGH as headaches in the presence of neck pain and pathology of the cervical spine, including disease related to bone, disc, and/or soft tissue [3]. The ICHD-3 diagnostic criteria require clinical and/or imaging evidence of cervical pathology (bone or soft tissue) and at least two of the following criteria: 1. temporal relation of headache onset and the spinal pathology; 2. headache improvement or resolution in parallel to improvement or resolution of spinal pathology; 3. reduced neck mobility and provocation of headache by stereotypical neck movements; 4. resolution of headaches after diagnostic cervical spine injections or associated nerve blocks [3].

These ICHD-3 criteria allow for a more standardized method of diagnosing CGH, however, given the relative lack of their use in prior publications, it is not surprising that there is tremendous variability in the reported rates of CGH prevalence. The estimated prevalence of CGH is reported to be 0.4–4% in the general population. However, in patients diagnosed with cervical pathology, greater than 85% may experience CGH, with a significant impact on patient morbidity, and quality of life [4–8]. Thus, given the high prevalence, and substantial influence on patient outcomes, it is imperative to formulate an understanding of the pathogenesis of CGH to develop appropriate treatment strategies.

3. Pathogenesis

The details of the pathogenesis of cervicogenic headaches remain elusive. As we review the current understanding of the pathogenesis of CGH, it is worth noting that most of the proposed theories rely on clinical findings and the underlying anatomic associations between the cervical spine and cranial nociceptive pathways. Although the origin of pain generators in the cervical spine remains speculative, neuroforaminal compression and uncovertebral joint arthropathy secondary to cervical spondylosis are likely contributors [6, 8–12]. There is some consensus regarding the transmission of the nociceptive stimulus from these potential pain generators. It is postulated that CGH are mediated through the convergence of nociceptive fibers from the upper cervical nerves (C1-C3) onto the trigeminal spinal nucleus, resulting in pain stimulus via the trigeminal afferents pathways [6, 8, 9, 13, 14]. This convergence of nociceptive stimuli can lead to the perception of fronto-temporal headaches and dysautonomia secondary to upper cervical spondylosis [8, 15].

The trigeminal afferent pathways are composed of three main nuclei and tracts: the mesencephalic nucleus and tract, the chief/principal sensory nucleus, and the spinal trigeminal nucleus and tract [16]. The spinal trigeminal tract conducts pain, temperature, and crude touch of the head, and is continuous caudally with the tract of Lissauer in the cervical spine. In the spine, the tract of Lissauer is formed by nociceptive fibers ascending and descending one to two levels in the dorsolateral white matter before entering the gray matter and decussating to join the ascending spinothalamic tract [17]. The convergence of the trigeminal spinal tract and the tract of Lissauer is a potential point of convergence between upper cervical spine (C1-C3) pain generators and ipsilateral CGH. However, this hypothesis cannot adequately explain cases of CGH in patients with spondylosis of the lower cervical spine [18, 19]. Several hypotheses have been proposed attempting to clarify the source of CGH from the lower cervical spine. One theory proposes that CGH are referred from the lower cervical spine by abnormal muscle and spinal kinematics caused by spondylosis [12, 20]. Cadaveric studies have demonstrated that the ligamentum nuchae and suboccipital muscles can be adherent to the occipital dura in a small subset of the population. This relationship could act as a mechanical conduit for the transformation of abnormal cervical spinal kinematics into nociceptive signals transferred to the dura in patients afflicted by spondylosis [15, 21]. Another theory postulates that aberrant connections between the spinal trigeminal tract and the spinothalamic tract could result in transmission of pain stimulus from the lower cervical region to the upper cervical region and ultimately perceived as fronto-temporal headaches [12, 20]. However, none of these theories have an adequate anatomical basis to clearly support their role in CGH. We hypothesize that CGH due to spondylosis of the lower cervical spine are likely referred through the sinuvertebral nerves (SVN) [6]. The SVN innervates the uncovertebral joints, the dura of the nerve root sleeve, and the nearby intervertebral discs. It travels mediolaterally from the uncovertebral joint towards the disc space in close association with the sympathetic and vascular plexus. Most notably, the SVN sends descending collaterals up to 3-disc spaces below its level of origin to communicate with the SVN of adjacent spinal levels (**Figure 1**). Thus, this anatomic pathway can account for neurovascular irritation in the lower cervical spine being referred to C1-C3 and in turn resulting in CGH [6]. The SVN plexus, cervical vasculature, and cervical nerve root are in proximity near the neural foramina that is formed by the uncovertebral joint, and facet joint (**Figure 1**). This region, coined the unco-vasculo-radicular (UVR) junction, is a likely candidate as a pain generator in CGH [6].

The SVN and neuroforaminal compression at the UVR junction do not adequately explain the associated dysautonomia that is commonly seen in CGH. However, autonomic pathways do connect the cervical plexus and the hypoglossal and vagal nerves through the C1 and C2 nerve roots. Moreover, C1-C4 are linked through the superior

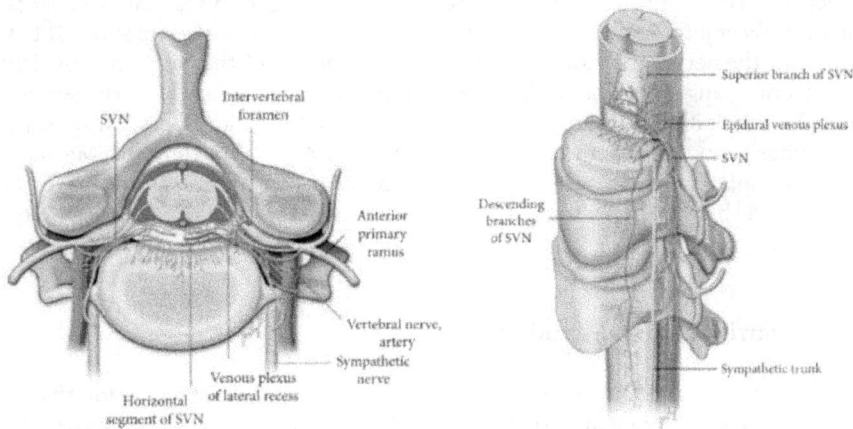

Figure 1.
Axial (left) and parasagittal (right) illustration of the course of the sinuvertebral nerve and its relationship to the ventral dura mater, nerve root, and sympathetic trunk.

cervical sympathetic ganglion (**Figure 1**). Thus, irritation of the dura, or nerve root sleeve in cervical spondylosis can cause aberrant activity in the sympathetic afferent pathways resulting in autonomic symptoms [6, 22].

Admittedly the pathogenesis of CGH is still not completely understood and is likely multifactorial, however, to date, no other hypothesis has laid out a clearer pathway for the cause of CGH due to spondylosis of the upper and lower cervical spine. To further clarify this theory, we will discuss the neurovascular anatomy of the SVN in the following section.

4. Relevant anatomy

The course of the sinuvertebral nerve (SVN) and sympathetic innervation of the cervical spine including the ventral dura, disc, and facet joints are essential to understanding the potential mechanism of CGH. The SVN plays a key role in the transmission of the pain in CGH [6].

The SVN, also known as the ramus meningismus or recurrent meningeal nerve of Luschka, was first described by Von Luschka in 1850 as he noted the nerve passing through the intervertebral foramen into the spinal canal and branches that remained outside of the dura mater. Its course was further revealed through cadaveric studies by Drs. Edgar and Nundy in the 1960's [23]. The SVN, a branch of the anterior primary ramus of the cervical nerve root, travels from outside the vertebral foramen, posterolateral to the uncovertebral joint, into the spinal canal where its middle branches innervate the ventral dura, posterior longitudinal ligament, and the intervertebral disc. Near its origin it receives fibers from the sympathetic trunk through the gray ramus communicantes. It also receives sympathetic input from the vertebral nerve which courses along the vertebral artery. The SVN has ascending and descending branches that traverse up to three vertebral levels [10]. Within the foramen and lateral recess there is a close relationship with the epidural venous plexus (**Figure 1**). This region is coined the unco-vasculo-radicular (UVR) junction, a narrow pathway where the SVN plexus, cervical vasculature, and the cervical nerve root join.

Potential sources of pain generation in cervicogenic headaches include paraspinal muscles, ligamentous injury, intervertebral disc, and spondylotic changes such as uncovertebral and facet arthropathy [22]. CGH is associated with tenderness of cervical paraspinal muscles and there are myofascial trigger points that can instigate pain [24]. Facet joint instability or hypertrophy at upper cervical segments (C1 to C3) can irritate the nerves that converge at the spinal segment of the trigeminal nucleus. Spondylotic changes and disc bulges throughout the rest of the cervical spine can lead to SVN irritation through compression at the UVR junction. Cervical stenosis and kyphosis can also generate pain from placing tension on the dura [6]. Mechanical traction on suboccipital tissues, the ligamentum nuchae and rectus posterior capitus minor muscle have been postulated to place tension on the dura which can lead to CGH [25, 26].

5. Differential diagnosis and work up

Cervicogenic headaches due to spondylosis are a diagnosis of exclusion that require physicians to rule out other intracranial and intraspinal pathologies such as neoplasms, tumors, inflammatory disease, and vascular pathologies. As previously mentioned, the ICHD-3 diagnostic criteria for CGH require clinical and/or imaging evidence of cervical pathology (bone or soft tissue) and at least two of the following criteria: 1. temporal relation of the onset of headache and the spinal pathology; 2. headache improvement or resolution in parallel to improvement or resolution of spinal pathology; 3. reduced neck mobility and provocation of headache by stereotypical neck movements; 4. resolution of headaches after diagnostic cervical spine injections or associated nerve blocks [3].

The differential diagnosis for CGH is broad, and frequently includes chronic paroxysmal headaches (CPH), C2 neuralgia, tension type headaches (TTH), and migraine headaches (MH). Differentiating CGH form these other entities can be challenging, and generally relies on symptomatology, presence of cervical pathology, and clinical response to treatment [6, 8, 27]. Patients with CGH typically experience 1 or 2 headaches per day, whereas those with CPH complain of more than 15 headaches daily; and unlike CGH, CPH patients report symptom relief with indomethacin therapy [1, 6]. C2 neuralgia presents with stereotypical pain in the occipital region and does not require the presence of unilateral neck pain often seen in CGH. Tension headaches can be bilateral, and MH can have side shifts, whereas CGH symptoms are usually unilateral on the side of the cervical pathology. Nausea/vomiting and photophobia can be present in both CGH and MH, however, their frequency and severity are much less pronounced in CGH as compared to MH. Moreover, MH symptoms may respond to ergotamine derivatives and sumatriptan whereas CGH symptoms do not [28–30].

Cervicogenic headaches typically present with episodic, and unilateral headaches that originate in the occipital area and generalize to involve fronto-temporal regions and the entire hemicranium. Unilaterality, without shifting of sides, is a hallmark presenting feature of CGH, although in severe cases bilateral symptoms have been reported [6, 31]. CGH patients will have associated radiculopathy such as pain, numbness, tingling, or weakness along the course of the involved nerve. They will often complain of reduced neck mobility. Finally, resolution of headaches after cervical and occipital nerve blocks is a defining feature of CGH.

As for radiographic features of CGH, there are no imaging characteristics that can assist in the differentiating CGH from other pathologies. Findings on computed tomography (CT), CT myelography, and magnetic resonance imaging (MRI) can include spondylosis, osteochondrosis, and disc osteophyte complex with foraminal or spinal stenosis; however, none of these features are unique to CGH [8, 32].

Neuro-interventional procedures such as intra-articular injections, nerve root blocks, and epidural injections can serve as both a diagnostic and therapeutic interventions [33, 34]. Bogduk et al. reported on 161 patients that were treated with cervical nerve root blocks and observed a reduction in CGH symptoms in 59% of patients [10]. Similarly, Persson et al. presented a series 275 consecutive patients with cervical radiculopathy and identified 161 with CGH. Following cervical nerve root blocks, 69% of the patients in this series reported relief from CGH symptoms [7]. These series highlight the value of neuro-interventional procedures in the armamentarium of clinicians for diagnosing and treating CGH.

6. Surgical management of cervicogenic headaches

The management of patients suffering from cervicogenic headaches is a challenging task and requires a multifaceted approach. The first steps in the treatment process involve medical therapies such as multimodal analgesia, physical therapy, and neuro-interventional procedures (e.g. intra-articular/epidural injections). If the patients' symptoms fail to respond to maximal medical therapies, surgical interventions may be considered if the headache is accompanied by other signs of radiculopathy [34, 35]. There are numerous reports in the literature attesting to successful and durable treatment of CGH with both anterior and posterior surgical approaches [6, 8, 36–40]. The common thread among the successful surgical treatments appears to be adequate decompression of the neurovascular structures at the unco-vasculo-radicular (UVR) junction. The anterior surgical approach is a minimally invasive technique that provides a direct route for ventral decompression of the UVR junction and addresses all of the potential nociceptive sources (e.g. disc, dura mater, posterior longitudinal ligament, foraminal stenosis) [38]. Conversely, the posterior approach relies on indirect decompression of the UVR junction dorsally and does not address the ventral nociceptive sources [38]. In following section we will review the existing literature for the posterior and anterior surgical techniques and describe the technical nuances of the anterior cervical surgical approach.

6.1 Posterior cervical decompressive surgery

The optimal surgical approach for the treatment of cervicogenic headaches remains controversial, with both anterior and posterior approaches reported to have an impact on symptom relief [41, 42]. Much of the surgical decision making still relies on clinical acumen and anecdotal surgeon experience, leading to variability in treatment paradigms [8, 37–39]. Despite this lack of consensus, there is some clinical evidence in support of posterior cervical decompressive surgery. Jansen et al. reported positive results on 8 patients that were successfully treated for CGH using posterior cervical laminoplasties. Six of the patients had complete relief of symptoms and 2 patients experienced improvement of their preoperative symptoms [38]. Although symptom relief appears to be considerable with posterior decompression, the durability of relief remains questionable. The durability of pain relief appears especially less pronounced as compared to the anterior approaches, with higher rates of delayed recurrence reported at 1 year [20]. Shimohata et al. noted that recurrence is typically less severe than the original symptoms and may be related to the disruption of the posterior cervical tension band resulting in abnormal spinal kinematics [20]. Similarly, Thind et al. theorized that a posterior approach can only achieve an indirect decompression of the UVR junction and fails to adequately address the irritation from the ventral dura mater and disc osteophytes [6]. Notwithstanding that the quality of the existing evidence is lacking, clinical trends appear to favor anterior cervical approaches in the treatment of CGH. Our group also advocates for the anterior cervical surgical approach when treating CGH. We believe that the anterior approach allows for a minimally invasive approach to the ventral spine, while preserving the posterior ligamentous and muscular tension band.

6.2 Anterior cervical decompressive surgery

The anterior cervical approach for addressing cervicogenic headaches is comprised of the anterior cervical discectomy and fusion (ACDF), and cervical disc arthroplasty (CDA). Similar to the posterior cervical approach, the literature on anterior approaches is heterogenous and difficult to generalize. However, there is convincing support for both ACDF and CDA in providing significant clinical relief of CGH symptoms. The anterior cervical discectomy and fusion is a well-established approach that has been applied to the treatment of CGH with favorable results. Jansen et al. presented a series of 51 patients treated with ACDF. Their results demonstrated 85% complete relief and 15% partial relief of CGH symptoms postoperatively [37]. Similarly, Liu et al. reported 34 patients undergoing ACDF with significant pain relief in all patients postoperatively [40]. Jansen et al. further demonstrated the long-term efficacy of ACDF when reporting 86% complete and 14% partial symptom relief in a series of 56 patients diagnosed with CGH [37–39]. This long-term relief of CGH symptoms after ACDF was again demonstrated when Schofferman et al. reported long term follow up (mean 37 months) for 9 patients with CGH and associated symptoms of nausea, arm pain, dizziness, and visual disturbances. Postoperatively 56% of patients reported complete relief of headaches and 44% reported partial relief. The mean Oswestry Disability Index for these patients significantly improved from 62 to 35, and all patients stated that they would choose to undergo the same surgery again to achieve similar outcomes [43].

Cervical disc arthroplasty is a contemporary addition to the surgical armamentarium of spine surgeons that allows for the preservation of spinal motion. Recent data suggests that CDA could provide longer lasting symptom relief than ACDF when treating CGH [4, 6, 35, 41]. Riina et al. performed a post hoc analysis of two randomized, controlled, multicenter clinical trials involving 1004 patients with CGH treated by ACDF or CDA [35]. Headaches were evaluated using the Neck Disability Index (NDI) questionnaire, with 865 (86.2%) patients complaining of headaches. Mild (grade 1, 2) headaches were reported in 342 patients (34.1%), and severe (grade 3, 4, 5) headaches were reported in 523 patients (52.1%). After the 24 months follow up period, 280 (34.9%) patients reported complete relief of headaches (grade 0), 375 (46.7%) patients reported mild headaches (grade 1 or 2), and 148 patients reported severe headaches (18.4%). The majority of both ACDF (58.5%) and CDA (64%) groups demonstrated statistically significant improvements from baseline symptoms at all time points during the follow up period. Notably, 13.7% of patients in the ACDF group and 8.4% in the CDA group experienced worsening headaches. Riina and colleagues concluded that CDA patients had more frequent improvements in headaches than patients treated with ACDF. However, they found no difference in headache scores, or in overall improvement of headache severity between the two groups at 24 months follow up [35]. Schrot et al. presented slightly different findings in a post hoc analysis of 260 patients treated with single-level ACDF or CDA followed for 24 months [36]. Eighty eight percent of patients reported baseline headaches, with 52% reporting severe headaches (NDI 3 or greater) preoperatively. Unlike the results from Riina et al., the authors found no significant differences in headache relief between ACDF and CDA groups. Interestingly, Schrot et al. noted that spinal pathology of the upper cervical spine was associated with greater preoperative headache scores, although the authors failed to show any correlation between the level of operation and post-operative headache scores [36]. Liu et al. performed a more nuanced analysis of patients that underwent single and two-level ACDF or CDA and evaluated headache response to each treatment [44]. For the single level group, after 60 months of follow up, both ACDF and CDA cohorts demonstrated similar statistically significant improvements in mean NDI headache scores. For the two-level groups both ACDF and CDA cohorts showed significant improvements from baseline headache scores, however, the CDA group demonstrated a greater magnitude of relief from baseline during early to moderate follow up period, although this difference disappeared after 18 months. Liu and colleagues concluded that both ACDF and CDA provide meaningful relief of cervicogenic headaches but highlighted a potential for higher degree of relief after two level CDA [44]. One explanation for the disappearance of the difference between ACDF and CDA over time may be the eventual progression of abnormal kinematics of the cervical spine [6]. Most recently, Thind et al. completed an exhaustive 7 year post hoc analysis of 437 patients that underwent one-level or two-level ACDF or CDA for symptomatic cervical spondylosis [6]. One hundred and eighty-five patients were identified for the one-level group and 252 patients in the two-level group. Approximately 50% of patients in the one-level and two-level groups reported NDI headache scores of 3 or greater at baseline. Results for both one level and two-level ACDF and CDA groups demonstrated statistically significant headache relief after 7 years of follow up. However, in contrast to findings by Liu et al. regarding two-level CDA, Thind et al. noticed a more profound improvement in headache scores in the CDA group as compared to ACDF patients at 7 year follow up. The authors concluded that relief from CGH is durable up to 7 years after both ACDF and CDA. To explain the observed superior long-term outcomes in the CDA group, Thind et al. emphasized the importance of the preservation of normal spinal kinematics resulting in a reduction of irritation at the UVR [6].

As demonstrated by the lack of consensus among authors, the optimal surgical option regarding ACDF or CDA remains complex and nuanced. However, reviewing the current literature reiterates the success of both anterior cervical approaches in the management of CGH, and supports the hypothesis of a ventral source for the pain generators (e.g. *dura*, disc, UVR zone). Ultimately, surgeon comfort and access to proper surgical equipment will dictate which approach is optimal.

6.3 Anterior cervical surgical technique

The anterior surgical corridor to the cervical spine has been a workhorse in the armamentarium of spine surgeons since the 1950's when first described by Robison, Smith, and Cloward [45, 46]. This approach allows for a minimally invasive technique to address ventral spinal pathology without the disruption of the posterior spinal tension band. In this section we will briefly review the critical steps in the anterior cervical approach for the decompression of the unco-vasculo-radicular junction in patients diagnosed with cervicogenic headaches.

After performing an appropriate surgical pause during which we administer antibiotics and steroids in non-diabetic patients, the patient is intubated, and proper vascular access is obtained. A standard supine position is used with the head slightly extended and firmly positioned in a foam ring. A small shoulder roll is inserted to allow for adequate extension and expansion of the surgical corridor. Care must be taken to avoid hyperextension or and rotation of the neck, especially if arthrodesis is planned. For access to the lower cervical levels, the shoulders may be taped down to allow for intraoperative visualization with fluoroscopy. External landmarks such as the hyoid bone (C3), thyroid bone (C4), or cricoid bone (C6) can be used to approximate the level of interest, however, we advocate for the use of fluoroscopy to ensure appropriate placement of the incision. We routinely approach the anterior cervical spine using a left sided approach, as there is some anecdotal evidence to suggest a lower risk of injury to the recurrent laryngeal nerve, however, either side is an acceptable choice [47–50]. If a redo operation is performed, care must be taken to approach from the same side as the prior surgery to avoid bilateral injury to the vagal nerve and vocal cord paralysis. The incision is placed in a transverse orientation extending from the midline to the medial border of the sternocleidomastoid muscle. Incorporating the incision within a skin crease results in the best cosmetic outcome. Our skin incision is typically 2–4 cm in length depending on the number of levels involved. Two to three mLs of Bupivacaine with 1:200,000 epinephrine is injected subcutaneously prior to skin incision. A scalpel is used to incise the dermis and a small self-retaining retractor is used to spread the soft tissue making the platysma muscle evident. Meticulous hemostasis is achieved at each tissue layer to avoid run down during surgery. Blunt dissection is used to spread the platysma, followed by monopolar cautery to cut through the muscle in a transverse orientation. Care must be taken to avoid injury to the vascular structures that run deep to the platysma. Aggressive subplatysmal dissection is used to allow for mobilization of the investing superficial cervical fascia. At this time, the sterno-cleidomastoid (SCM) muscle is identified laterally, and the cervical strap muscles are identified medially. The carotid artery is palpated and identified early on and kept lateral to the plane of dissection. An avascular tissue plane is developed bluntly between the SCM and the cervical strap muscles. This dissection is carried through the pre-tracheal fascia and continued medially towards the pre-vertebral fascia and the ventral spine. The longus coli muscles and the intervertebral discs are identified at this time, and a clamp is placed on the suspected disc space. Intraoperative fluoroscopy is used to confirm the level of interest. With the use of hand-held Cloward retractors, the longus coli muscles are elevated laterally using a subperiosteal technique as to avoid injury to the sympathetic cervical plexus. Self-retaining retractors are inserted deep to the longus coli muscles to retract the esophagus medially and the carotid sheath laterally. Distraction pins may be used if the disc space is collapsed, but care must be taken to avoid over distraction and injury to the posterior spinal elements. Using the microscope, a complete discectomy is performed followed by posterior longitudinal ligament resection, and bilateral unco-foraminotomies.

For arthrodesis, many different interbody and plating systems are available that allow for similar rates of arthrodesis. Meticulous care must be taken to decorticate the end plates and remove any disc material to maximize the chance of successful arthrodesis. However, one must avoid overzealous disruption of the endplates as this would increase the risk of subsidence. After placement of the interbody and screws intraoperative fluoroscopy is utilized to confirm appropriate placement of the implants.

As with arthrodesis, disc arthroplasty can be achieved with a variety of different artificial disc systems. At our institution, we have used the Mobi-C Cervical Disc (Zimmer Biomet, Westminster, Colorado) with good results. The preservation of the endplates is extremely important for arthroplasty as subsidence can lead to reduced range of motion and inadvertent arthrodesis. Moreover, the positioning of the artificial disc is of utmost importance, and intraoperative fluoroscopy is utilized to ensure the disc is midline and recessed appropriately inside the disc space. After adequate placement of the artificial disc, we apply a small amount of bone wax to the ventral surface of the adjacent vertebral bodies to reduce the risk for heterotopic ossification.

Upon completion of instrumentation, hemostasis is achieved, and the platysma and the dermis are reapproximated.

7. Conclusion

Cervicogenic headaches are a debilitating pathology that can cause a significant burden on patient quality of life. Given the relatively recent recognition of cervicogenic headaches, there remains considerable controversy regarding the underlying pathogenesis and optimal treatment strategies. There is a clear need for further research aimed at identifying the underlying pain generators in cervicogenic headaches. Moreover, high quality clinical trials are necessary to discern between treatment options. Importantly, medical management should be exhausted for headache control and headaches alone should not be the reason for recommending surgery. The anterior cervical surgical approach is a minimally invasive technique that has demonstrated promising results in relieving symptoms related to cervicogenic headaches and should be considered in the appropriate patient population.

Acknowledgements

Figure 1 courtesy of Neurospine Journal.

Disclosures

The corresponding author receives royalties and is a consultant for Zimmer Biomet.

Abbreviations

ACDF	anterior cervical discectomy and fusion
CDA	cervical disc arthroplasty
CGH	cervicogenic headaches
CPH	chronic paroxysmal headaches
ICHD-3	International Headache Society's Headache classification (ICHD-3)
MH	migraine headaches
SCM	sternocleidomastoid
SVN	sinuvertebral Nerves
TTH	tension type headaches
UVR	unco-vasculo-radicular (UVR)

Author details

Amir Goodarzi, Edwin Kulubya, Tejas Karnati and Kee Kim*
University of California Davis Department of Neurological Surgery,
Sacramento, USA

*Address all correspondence to: kdkim@ucdavis.edu

IntechOpen

References

[1] O. Sjaastad, C. Saunte, H. Hovdahl, H. Breivik, E. Grønbâk, "Cervicogenic" headache. An hypothesis, Cephalalgia. 3 (1983) 249-256. https://doi.org/10.1046/j.1468-2982.1983.0304249.x.

[2] O. Sjaastad, Cervicogenic headache the controversial headache, Clinical Neurology and Neurosurgery. 94 (1992) 147-149. https://doi.org/10.1016/0303-8467(92)90053-6.

[3] J. Olesen, Headache Classification Committee of the International Headache Society (IHS) The International Classification of Headache Disorders, 3rd edition, Cephalalgia. 38 (2018) 1-211. https://doi.org/10.1177/0333102417738202.

[4] J. Riina, P.A. Anderson, L.T. Holly, K. Flint, K.E. Davis, K.D. Riew, The effect of an anterior cervical operation for cervical radiculopathy or myelopathy on associated headaches, Journal of Bone and Joint Surgery - Series A. 91 (2009) 1919-1923. https://doi.org/10.2106/JBJS.H.00500.

[5] R.J. Schrot, J.S. Mathew, Y. Li, L. Beckett, H.W. Bae, K.D. Kim, Headache relief after anterior cervical discectomy: Post hoc analysis of a randomized investigational device exemption trial: Clinical article, Journal of Neurosurgery: Spine. 21 (2014) 217-222. https://doi.org/10.3171/2014.4.SPINE13669.

[6] H. Thind, D. Ramanathan, J. Ebinu, D. Copenhaver, K.D. Kim, Headache relief is maintained 7 years after anterior cervical spine surgery: Post hoc analysis from a multicenter randomized clinical trial and cervicogenic headache hypothesis, Neurospine. 17 (2020) 365-373. https://doi.org/10.14245/ns.2040004.002.

[7] L.C.G. Persson, J.Y. Carlsson, L. Anderberg, Headache in patients with cervical radiculopathy: A prospective study with selective nerve root blocks in 275 patients, European Spine Journal. 16 (2007) 953-959. https://doi.org/10.1007/s00586-006-0268-8.

[8] S. Haldeman, S. Dagenais, Cervicogenic headaches: A critical review, Spine Journal. 1 (2001) 31-46. https://doi.org/10.1016/S1529-9430(01)00024-9.

[9] C.R. Hunter, F.H. Mayfield, Role of the upper cervical roots in the production of pain in the head, The American Journal of Surgery. 78 (1949) 743-751. https://doi.org/10.1016/0002-9610(49)90316-5.

[10] N. Bogduk, M. Windsor, A. Inglis, The innervation of the cervical intervertebral discs, Spine. 13 (1988) 2-8. https://doi.org/10.1097/00007632-198801000-00002.

[11] M.A. Edgar, S. Nundy, Innervation of the spinal dura mater, BMJ Publishing Group, 1966. https://www.ncbi.nlm.nih.gov/pmc/articles/PMC496104/ (accessed October 5, 2020).

[12] N. Bogduk, Cervicogenic headache: anatomic basis and pathophysiologic mechanisms., Current Pain and Headache Reports. 5 (2001) 382-386. https://doi.org/10.1007/s11916-001-0029-7.

[13] F.W.L. Kerr, R.A. Olafson, Trigeminal and Cervical Volleys: Convergence on Single Units in the Spinal Gray at C-1 and C-2, Archives of Neurology. 5 (1961) 171-178. https://doi.org/10.1001/archneur.1961.00450140053005.

[14] F.W.L. Kerr, Central relationships of trigeminal and cervical primary afferents in the spinal cord and medulla, Brain Research.

43 (1972) 561-572. https://doi.
org/10.1016/0006-8993(72)90408-8.

[15] M.E. Alix, D.K. Bates, A proposed
etiology of cervicogenic headache: The
neurophysiologic basis and anatomic
relationship between the dura mater
and the rectus posterior capitis minor
muscle, Journal of Manipulative and
Physiological Therapeutics. 22 (1999)
534-539. https://doi.org/10.1016/
S0161-4754(99)70006-0.

[16] S. Price, D.T. Daly, Neuroanatomy,
Trigeminal Nucleus, StatPearls
Publishing, 2020. http://www.ncbi.nlm.
nih.gov/pubmed/30969645 (accessed
October 12, 2020).

[17] D. Purves, G.J. Augustine, D.
Fitzpatrick, L.C. Katz, A.-S. LaMantia,
J.O. McNamara, S.M. Williams, Central
Pain Pathways: The Spinothalamic
Tract, (2001). https://www.ncbi.nlm.
nih.gov/books/NBK10967/ (accessed
October 12, 2020).

[18] G. Gondo, T. Watanabe, J. Kawada,
M. Tanaka, K. Yamamoto, S. Tanaka, S.
Endo, A case of cervicogenic headache
caused by C5 nerve root derived
shwannoma: Case report, Cephalalgia.
37 (2017) 902-905. https://doi.
org/10.1177/0333102416658713.

[19] R. -P Michler, G. Bovim, O. Sjaastad,
Disorders in the Lower Cervical Spine.
A Cause of Unilateral Headache? A
Case Report, Headache: The Journal of
Head and Face Pain. 31 (1991) 550-551.
https://doi.org/10.1111/j.1526-4610.1991.
hed3108550.x.

[20] K. Shimohata, K. Hasegawa, O.
Onodera, M. Nishizawa, T. Shimohata,
The Clinical Features, Risk Factors, and
Surgical Treatment of Cervicogenic
Headache in Patients With Cervical
Spine Disorders Requiring Surgery,
Headache. 57 (2017) 1109-1117. https://
doi.org/10.1111/head.13123.

[21] B.S. Mitchell, B.K. Humphreys,
E. O'Sullivan, Attachments of the
ligamentum nuchae to cervical posterior
spinal dura and the lateral part of the
occipital bone., Journal of Manipulative
and Physiological Therapeutics. 21
(1998) 145-8. http://www.ncbi.nlm.nih.
gov/pubmed/9567232.

[22] K. Kim, Kee; Ramanathan,
Dinesh; Provoast, Cervicogenic
Headache - Review of Pathogenesis and
Management, Journal of Neurosurgery
Imaging and Techniques. 3 (2018)
193-196.

[23] S. Edgar, MA; Nundy, Innervation
of the spinal dura mater, J Neurol
Neurosurg Psychiatry. (1966) 530-534.

[24] B.J. Freund, M. Schwartz,
Treatment of whiplash associated with
neck pain with botulinum toxin-A: A
pilot study, Journal of Rheumatology. 27
(2000) 481-484.

[25] M.E. Alix, D.K. Bates, A proposed
etiology of cervicogenic headache: The
neurophysiologic basis and anatomic
relationship between the dura mater
and the rectus posterior capitis minor
muscle, Journal of Manipulative and
Physiological Therapeutics. 22 (1999)
534-539. https://doi.org/10.1016/
S0161-4754(99)70006-0.

[26] B.S. Mitchell, B.K. Humphreys,
E. O'Sullivan, Attachments of the
ligamentum nuchae to cervical posterior
spinal dura and the lateral part of the
occipital bone., Journal of Manipulative
and Physiological Therapeutics. 21
(1998) 145-148.

[27] N. Bogduk, J. Govind, Cervicogenic
headache: an assessment of the evidence
on clinical diagnosis, invasive tests, and
treatment, The Lancet Neurology. 8
(2009) 959-968. https://doi.org/10.1016/
S1474-4422(09)70209-1.

[28] O. Sjaastad, G. Bovim, L.J. Stovner,
Lateralitly of pain and other migraine
criteria in common migraine. A
comparison with cervicogenic headache,
Functional Neurology. 7 (1992) 289-294.

[29] O. Sjaastad, T. Fredriksen, J.A. Pareja, A. Stolt-Nielsen, M. Vincent, Coexistence of cervicogenic headache and migraine without aura (?), Functional Neurology. 14 (1999) 209-218.

[30] O. Sjaastad, G. Bovim, Cervicogenic headache. The differentiation from common migraine. An overview, Functional Neurology. 6 (1991) 93-100.

[31] N. Merskey, H; Bogduk, Classification of Chronic Pain, Classification of Chronic Pain. IASP Press, Seattle. (1994).

[32] T.A. Fredriksen, R. Fougner, A. Tangerud, O. Sjaastad, Cervicogenic Headache. Radiological Investigations Concerning Head/Neck, Cephalalgia. 9 (1989) 139-146. https://doi. org/10.1046/j.1468-2982.1989.0902139.x.

[33] N. Bogduk, The clinical anatomy of the cervical dorsal rami, Spine. 7 (1982) 319-330. https://doi. org/10.1097/00007632-198207000-00001.

[34] E. Wang, D. Wang, Treatment of Cervicogenic Headache with Cervical Epidural Steroid Injection, Current Pain and Headache Reports. 18 (2014). https://doi.org/10.1007/s11916-014-0442-3.

[35] J. Riina, P.A. Anderson, L.T. Holly, K. Flint, K.E. Davis, K.D. Riew, The Effect of an Anterior Cervical Operation for Cervical Radiculopathy or Myelopathy on Associated Headaches, The Journal of Bone and Joint Surgery-American Volume. 91 (2009) 1919-1923. https://doi.org/10.2106/JBJS.H.00500.

[36] R.J. Schrot, J.S. Mathew, Y. Li, L. Beckett, H.W. Bae, K.D. Kim, Headache relief after anterior cervical discectomy: Post hoc analysis of a randomized investigational device exemption trial: Clinical article, Journal of Neurosurgery: Spine. 21 (2014)

217-222. https://doi.org/10.3171/2014.4. SPINE13669.

[37] J. Jansen, Surgical treatment of non-responsive cervicogenic headache, Clin Exp Rheumatol. 18(2 Suppl (n.d.) S67-70.

[38] J. Jansen, Laminoplasty--a possible treatment for cervicogenic headache? Some ideas on the trigger mechanism of CeH, Funct Neurol. 14(3) (n.d.) 163-5.

[39] J. Jansen, Surgical treatment of cervicogenic headache, Cephalalgia. 28 (2008) 41-44. https://doi. org/10.1111/j.1468-2982.2008.01620.x.

[40] H. Liu, A. Ploumis, S. Wang, C. Li, H. Li, Treatment of Cervicogenic Headache Concurrent with Cervical Stenosis by Anterior Cervical Decompression and Fusion, Clinical Spine Surgery. 30 (2017) E1093–E1097. https://doi.org/10.1097/BSD.0000000000000291.

[41] H.C. Diener, M. Kaminski, G. Stappert, D. Stolke, B. Schoch, Lower cervical disc prolapse may cause cervicogenic headache: Prospective study in patients undergoing surgery, Cephalalgia. 27 (2007) 1050-1054. https://doi. org/10.1111/j.1468-2982.2007.01385.x.

[42] J. Jansen, E. Markakis, B. Rama, J.J. Hildebrandt CEPHALALGIA Jansen, H.J. Hemicranial, J. Jansen, E. Markakis, B. Rama, Hemicranial attacks or permanent hemicrania-a sequel of upper cervical root compression, n.d.

[43] J. Schofferman, K. Garges, N. Goldthwaite, M. Koestler, E. Libby, Upper cervical anterior diskectomy and fusion improves discogenic cervical headaches, Spine. 27 (2002) 2240-2244. https://doi.org/10.1097/00007632-200210150-00011.

[44] J.J. Liu, G. Cadena, R.R. Panchal, R.J. Schrot, K.D. Kim, Relief of

Cervicogenic Headaches after Single-Level and Multilevel Anterior Cervical Diskectomy: A 5-Year Post Hoc Analysis, Global Spine Journal. 6 (2016) 563-570. https://doi.org/10.1055/s-0035-1570086.

[45] R.B. Cloward, The anterior approach for removal of ruptured cervical disks., Journal of Neurosurgery. 15 (1958) 602-617. https://doi.org/10.3171/jns.1958.15.6.0602.

[46] R.A. Robinson, G.W. Smith, Anterolateral cervical disc removal and interbody fusion for cervical disc syndrome, SAS Journal. 4 (2010) 34-35. https://doi.org/10.1016/j.esas.2010.01.003.

[47] M. Miscusi, A. Bellitti, S. Peschillo, F.M. Polli, P. Missori, R. Delfini, Does recurrent laryngeal nerve anatomy condition the choice of the side for approaching the anterior cervical spine?, Journal of Neurosurgical Sciences. 51 (2007) 61-4. http://www.ncbi.nlm.nih.gov/pubmed/17571036.

[48] A.M. Thomas, D.K. Fahim, J.M. Gemechu, Anatomical Variations of the Recurrent Laryngeal Nerve and Implications for Injury Prevention during Surgical Procedures of the Neck., Diagnostics (Basel, Switzerland). 10 (2020). https://doi.org/10.3390/diagnostics10090670.

[49] A. Arantes, S. Gusmão, F. Rubinstein, R. Oliveira, Microsurgical anatomy of the recurrent laryngeal nerve: Applications on the anterior approach to the cervical spine, Arquivos de Neuro-Psiquiatria. 62 (2004) 707-710. https://doi.org/10.1590/s0004-282x2004000400026.

[50] N.A. Ebraheim, J. Lu, M. Skie, B.E. Heck, R.A. Yeasting, Vulnerability of the recurrent laryngeal nerve in the anterior approach to the lower cervical spine, in: Spine, Spine (Phila Pa 1976), 1997: pp. 2664-2667. https://doi.org/10.1097/00007632-199711150-00015.

Chapter 2

The Cervical Hybrid Arthroplasty

Pablo Pazmiño

Abstract

The cervical hybrid arthroplasty is a surgical option for appropriately indicated patients, and high success rates have been reported in the literature. Complications and failures are often associated with patient indications or technical variables, and the goal of this chapter is to assist surgeons in understanding these factors.

Keywords: cervical hybrid arthroplasty, cervical disc arthroplasty, disc replacement, artificial disc replacement (ADR), cervical artificial disc replacement (C-ADR), anterior cervical discectomy and fusion (ACDF), radiculopathy, myelopathy, cervical degenerative disc disease, cervical disc herniation, herniated disc

1. Introduction

Spine surgeons and patients together are confronted with several surgical options when managing cervical pains which have not responded to conservative treatment options. Multilevel cervical disc pathology is defined as two or more segments of the cervical spine that have herniated, or degenerated, which are subsequently causing significant axial pain with radiculopathy, resulting in disability and a loss of productivity. Anterior cervical discectomy and fusion (ACDF) is considered the gold standard treatment for multilevel cervical spondylosis. However there are some long term drawbacks involving the development of subsidence, pseudarthrosis and the degeneration of adjacent segments [1–4]. Cervical artificial disc replacement (C-ADR) has been demonstrated to be a safe and effective means of treating single-level or multilevel cervical disc pathology by several prospective studies from the United States Food and Drug Administration and by some meta-analyses [5–11]. In patients who have multilevel pathology, there is a growing enthusiasm towards definitive management in the form of a cervical hybrid arthroplasty [12–15]. The cervical hybrid arthroplasty is a procedure wherein an artificial disc replacement can be placed at one level, with a cervical fusion device implanted at another nearby injured disc (**Figure 1**).

2. Methodology

2.1 Indications

While indications for both fusions and arthroplasty are always in a state of flux certain considerations can be made to this point. Both implants share similar clinical goals of decreased pain with increased function, and therefore there is considerable overlap in regards to their surgical indications. As a general rule both fusions and arthroplasty can be indicated for any skeletally mature patient who has neck pain and/or radiculopathy which has failed a course of six weeks of conservative nonoperative therapy.

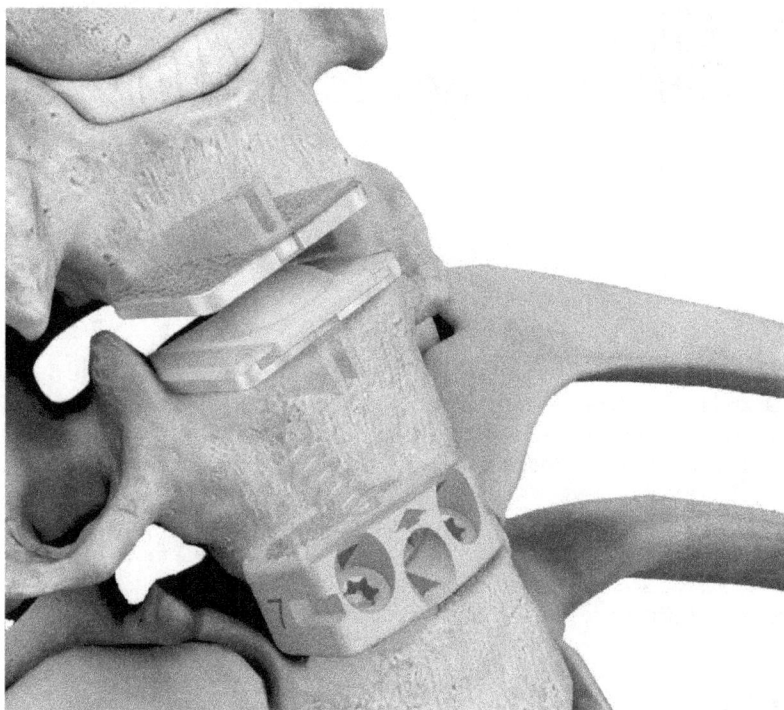

Figure 1.
The cervical hybrid arthroplasty.

Nonoperative treatments vary among medication, therapy, traction, chiropractic, acupuncture, activity modification, epidural injections and pain management.
    Cervical hybrid arthroplasty Inclusion Criteria:

- Has cervical disc pathology at two [2] cervical levels (from C3 C7) requiring surgical treatment and involving intractable radiculopathy, neck pain and/or myelopathy.

- Has a herniated disc and/or osteophyte formation at each level to be treated that is producing symptomatic nerve root and/or spinal cord compression. The pathology correlates directly with documented findings on patient history and exam (e.g., neck pain with arm pain, functional deficit and/or neurological deficit), and the requirement for surgical treatment is confirmed by imaging studies (e.g., MRI, CT, x-rays, etc.).

- Has the presence of progressive symptoms or signs of nerve root/spinal cord compression despite continued non-operative management.

- Has no prior surgical intervention at the involved levels or any subsequent planned/staged surgical procedure at the involved or adjacent level(s).

- The cervical disc arthroplasty implant can be considered for symptomatic patients within the earlier stages of disc pathology, prior to bony collapse and significant spurring in order to limit postoperative heterotopic ossification.

- Must be at least 18 years of age and be skeletally mature at the time of surgery

2.2 Contraindications

Often with cervical pathology a fusion based implant is warranted, so for the purpose of this chapter we will set our focus on contraindications specific to the arthroplasty implant.

- Advanced abnormal changes such as bony collapse at the proposed surgery level.

- Advanced degeneration or trauma to the facet joints on the back of the spine.

- An active systemic infection or infection at the surgical site.

- An unnatural shape (e.g. hyperkyphosis deformity, hyperlordosis deformity) of the neck.

- A known allergy to titanium, stainless steel, polyurethane, polyethylene or ethylene oxide residuals.

- A known allergy to PEEK, ceramic, or the given implants requisite metallurgy.

- Has documented or diagnosed cervical instability relative to adjacent segments at either level, defined by dynamic (flexion/extension) radiographs showing:

- Sagittal plane translation >3.5 mm, or

- Sagittal plane angulation >20°;

- Has severe pathology of the facet joints of the involved vertebral bodies.

- Has been previously diagnosed with osteopenia or osteomalacia.

- Has been previously diagnosed with diagnosis of osteoporosis.

- If the level of bone mineral density is a T score of −1.5 or lower.

- Has presence of spinal metastases.

- Has overt or active bacterial infection, either local or systemic.

- Has chronic or acute renal failure or prior history of renal disease.

- Has received drugs or therapies that may interfere with bone metabolism within two weeks prior to the planned date of spinal surgery (e.g., chemotherapy, radiation, steroids or methotrexate), excluding routine perioperative anti-inflammatory drugs.

- Has a history of an endocrine or metabolic disorder known to affect osteogenesis (e.g., Paget's Disease, renal osteodystrophy, Ehlers-Danlos Syndrome, or osteogenesis imperfecta).

- Has a condition that requires postoperative medications that interfere with the stability of the implant, such as steroids, chemotherapy, or radiation. (This does not include low-dose aspirin for prophylactic anticoagulation and routine perioperative anti-inflammatory drugs).

- Has a history of heterotopic ossification [16, 17].

- Has a history of a prior failed or delayed fusion at the proposed arthroplasty level.

3. Implants

3.1 Arthroplasty implants

Since 1955 there have been several accounts of a variety of implants which were the harbinger of the modern day cervical arthroplasty. Initial reports of disc replacements ranged from methylmethacrylate injections to unconstrained spheres composed of various substances ranging from silicone, rubber, and stainless steel [18–20]. Early arthroplasty designs never achieved much in the form of widespread practical application as they were forsaken after sparse clinical use. However, early success with lumbar disc replacements ushered in a new era of spinal arthroplasty in the cervical spine. In 1991 the Bristol/Cummins disc is credited as the first of the modern articulating Cervical Artificial Disc Replacement (C-ADR) devices which was implanted in 20 patients and was reported to be functional in several for as long as 12 years postoperatively [21]. Since then an array of designs have flooded the marketplace with materials ranging from metal-on-metal, metal-on-plastic, non-articulating metal bonded to plastic, plastic embedded in cloth, polymer fibers wound around a polycarbonate urethane core, and PEEK on PEEK [17, 22–24]. Despite a wide array of designs and formulations, manufacturers have been unable to emulate and reproduce the mechanical and load bearing properties of the innate human disc. Therefore the various axial and shear loads are still being transferred to the index and neighboring adjacent levels. In order to offset these loads different bearing designs have been conceived, each of which vary based on the amount of impedance, restraint and stability they confer to the spinal unit and dorsal facet joints. Implants without any mechanical impedance built in are considered unconstrained and allow for significant mobility while sacrificing some implant stability. Constrained devices impede movement of the spinal unit within the range of normal physiologic motion and infer greater implant stability by removing shear forces on the facet joints, but in turn place significant stress on the surfaces at the vertebral endplate-implant junction. Semiconstrained implants allow motion just outside the physiologic norm in effort to theoretically decrease the mechanical stresses felt at both at the facet joints and the interface between the implant and the bony surfaces. While often successful, these varied designs have also brought with them a concomitant range of complications with documented occurrences of extrusions, heterotopic ossification, osteolysis, and hardware failure [16, 23, 25–28].

3.2 Fusion implants

Following implantation of the disc replacement a successful cervical hybrid arthroplasty is conditional upon a solid foundation in the form of the adjacent fusion. Fusion implants can be grouped into stand alone versus standard plate and interbody cage designs. Often Allograft, Carbon fiber, Polyetheretherketone (PEEK), and titanium (Ti) have been designated for interbody cage designs. Each material varies in regards to their unique biocompatibility, surface topography, osseointegration, and imaging characteristics. Some implant manufacturers are also borrowing traits from other designs in efforts to improve upon attributes they lack. For example some designers are taking the once inert PEEK cage and bio-actively coating them with either Hydroxyapatite (HA) or Ti, creating a composite design in efforts to improve osseous integration.

4. Surgical rationale and decision making

4.1 Implant placement and rationale

The cervical hybrid arthroplasty provides the unique opportunity where with one procedure the surgeon can address an area of junctional kyphosis while simultaneously preserving motion at a neighboring disc. When considering all scenarios for a cervical hybrid surgery, there should be a consistent rationale in regards to which level to fuse and in which level to place the arthroplasty.

For the most part there are some straightforward scenarios which dictate which level warrants the cervical fusion implant. If one disc is entirely collapsed, demonstrates significant bony spurs, and/or heterotopic ossification, this level would assuredly justify the fusion implant. If the operative level lies within the inferior aspect of the spine (i.e. Cervical 6–7, C7-T1) sufficient reasoning exists towards the insertion of a fusion spacer at this level as opposed to an arthroplasty. This is because along the inferior limb of the cervical spine, the sub adjacent interspace levels are morphologically larger and well documented as demonstrating less motion [29–31]. Their size and innate stiffness coupled with the stability conferred by their adjoining anatomy makes these levels are ideally suited towards forming the foundation of the hybrid construct and bearing any subsequent transferred loads [31–33]. By contrast, the interspaces along the more cephalad aspect of the spine (Cervical 2–3, Cervical 3–4) routinely comprise a smaller footprint and consequently can only accommodate a smaller implant. As a result these smaller interspaces are often ideally suited towards fusion spacers which tend to come in more sizes and options. Furthermore if there is any indication of ongoing myelopathy or an underlying contiguous myelomalacia, this level would best be served with a fusion implant which would provide a stable postoperative environment. Otherwise in patients who have myelopathy only those without instability and symptoms due to soft disc herniations with or without minor spurs would be good candidates for an arthroplasty.

The core principle behind all arthroplasties is their perceived objective, once implanted, towards minimizing the biomechanical stresses placed on adjacent levels. With this in mind deciding which level should obtain the arthroplasty device is of paramount importance. As a rule of thumb, all efforts are geared towards placing the arthroplasty at the top of the overall construct in order to minimize stress at the superior neighboring and often more mobile disc [29, 34]. When this is not possible, in a circumstance where there are three disc herniations and the decision has been made only to operate on two of the discs because they are the only symptomatic levels, then the arthroplasty should be placed at the level nearest the third disc in hopes of preventing it from further deterioration. Studies have shown that the arthroplasty implant would limit transmission of angular, horizontal, and translation forces experienced by the adjacent third level disc [35–40].

4.2 Sequence of implantation

The sequence of implantation should be considered well in advance during the preoperative planning phase in order to limit complications. During insertion, tapping of the implants with the mallet can lead to an aggravation of an underlying stenotic area, or the migration and loosening of a previously inserted prosthesis [41, 42]. In order to avoid this for all cervical hybrid arthroplasty procedures a thorough decompression of all the intended disc spaces should be performed prior to any implant insertion, with priority given to the most stenotic level. In all circumstances the C-ADR should be implanted prior to the ACDF portion of the procedure. If implanting more than one arthroplasty, all trialing, rasping, drilling for both prostheses should be performed prior to C-ADR implantation [41, 43].

5. Surgical technique and pearls

5.1 Patient positioning

Patients commonly notice posterior neck pain following disc arthroplasty. The pain can be a result of surgical positioning, intraoperative distraction on the facet joints and capsules, or an indirect distraction on the endplates from the implant itself. Often these implants are inserted with a considerable amount of force so in order to limit the unsupported transfer of these forces to the paraspinal musculature and facet joints, a properly contoured support should be placed along the posterior aspect of the neck (**Figure 2a**).

5.2 Surgical approach and discectomy

The cervical hybrid arthroplasty is performed in the supine position under general anesthesia. A transverse incision in line with the planned arthroplasty level is employed for two- or three- level hybrid procedures (**Figure 2a**). Alternatively a longitudinal incision can be used for a more extensive procedure such as a multilevel procedure requiring corpectomies at the fusion level. Implantation of the arthroplasty always demands optimal visualization and therefore the incision should be inline with the proposed arthroplasty interspace while taking into consideration both the trajectory needed and the requisite instrumentation (**Figure 2b**). With that in mind following the skin incision, a standard Anterior Smith Robinson approach provides sufficient access to whichever interspace the surgeon plans to address first. After complete discectomy the endplates are denuded of all cartilaginous tissue with curettage prior to removal of any posterior uncinates or bone spurs. Prior to its removal the posterior longitudinal ligament is inspected for any tears or defects, which may give rise to sequestered fragments causing impingement on the thecal sac or neuroforamina. Once the discectomy has been performed care should be taken to remove any anterior or posterior osteophytes in order to contour the interspace inline with the proposed implant, and in doing so ensure a secure fit.

5.3 Measuring intraoperative depth

The width and depth of the intended arthroplasty can be assessed prior to even selecting a trial with the placement of an intraoperative ruler (**Figure 3a, b, Video 1**). Predetermination of the dimensions of the trial for the arthroplasty can easily be attained in this manner and thereby avoids catastrophic implant or trial related complications and consequences [42].

5.4 Midline placement

During a cervical hybrid arthroplasty the C-ADR implant should routinely be placed first so no adjacent plate or hardware obstructs any anatomic or fluoroscopic visualization. In order to secure proper midline positioning during intraoperative placement some arthroplasty implants have instrumentation designed to help verify

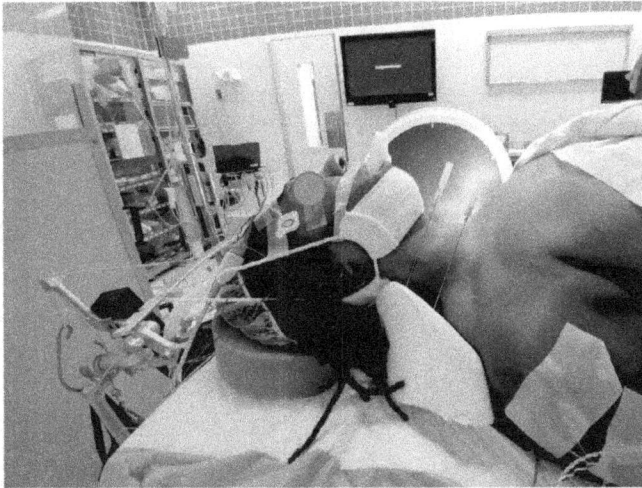

(a)

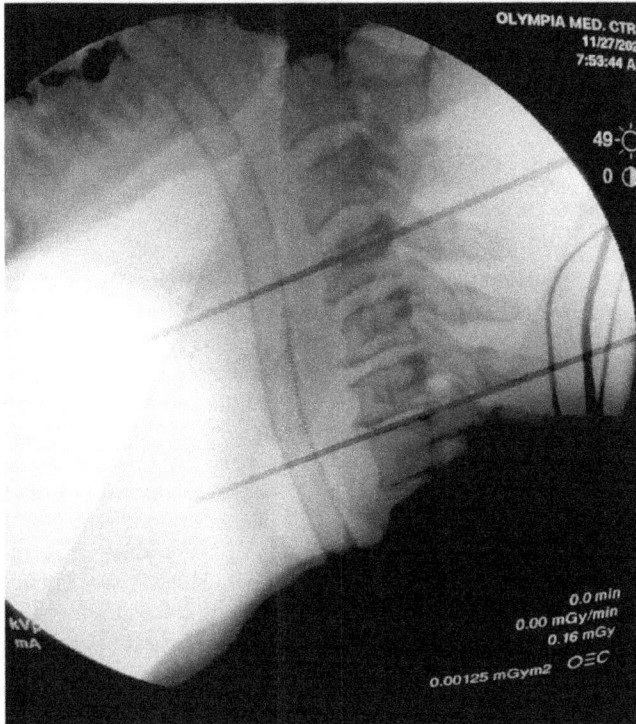

(b)

Figure 2.
(a) The cervical spine is supported here with a foam cushioned pillow, often used by the anesthesiologists when placing the patients in a prone position. In this case the foam cushion supports the neck by acting as a counter force to any horizontal translational or shear forces at play during final implant tapping and placement. Here a cervical bite block is used and a 10 lb. weight allows for axial traction through a neck holster. During surgery this same neck holster can be pulled by the anesthesiologist to allow indirect distraction of the interspace and therefore ease placement of the prosthesis and fusion spacers intraoperatively. The C-arm, pictured here, is left in the lateral position for the majority of the case. (b) Coincidentally the cushion also provides a stable surface where needles can be placed to confirm the length of the surgical incision for a longitudinal skin incision preoperatively.

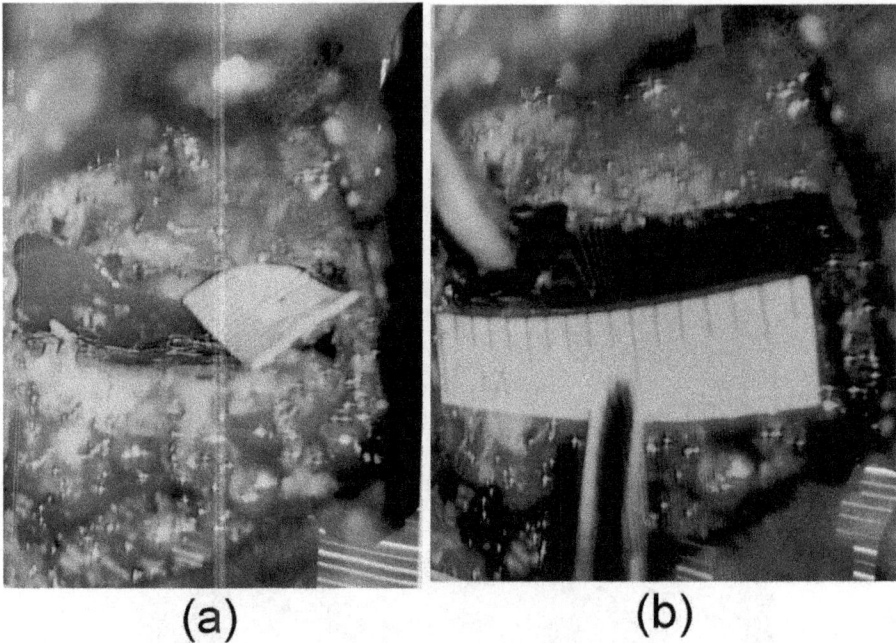

Figure 3.
(a) A standard ruler is cut to 16 mm and this ruler can then be placed within the interspace to evaluate the depth of the trial, and therefore implant needed. (b) This ruler can then be placed within the interspace to evaluate the width of the trial, and therefore implant needed.

the ideal location. This is important because minimizing prosthetic deviation to within 1.2 mm of the ideal center midline position, has been shown to ensure no detrimental clinical outcomes or long term repercussions [44]. In order to secure proper midline positioning first a collinear Anterior Posterior (AP) fluoroscopic view must be secured in line with the intended interspace (**Figure 4**). Once an appropriate image has been obtained, accurate midline positioning of the prosthesis can be confirmed (**Figure 5a-c**). In order to confirm proper midline positioning attention should be made towards discrete morphological and anatomical landmarks. First with visual inspection, confirming equidistant placement of the trial in regards to the longus coli. On fluoroscopy the spinous processes should lie en face and midline with respect to their corresponding vertebral bodies. The edges of the trial should lie equidistant with respect to each of the ascending bilateral uncinate joints. Final midline placement can be confirmed with fluoroscopic visualization (**Figure 5a**).

5.5 Measuring fluoroscopic depth

Most implant trials come with a drill, chisel, or similar device used to cut grooves in the vertebral body for insertion of the final implant. In order to confirm final implant placement the final imaging obtained while trialing can be compared with the spinal implant to confirm final and accurate positioning (**Figure 6a-c**).

5.6 Final implantation

After midline confirmation under fluoroscopy of the arthroplasty attention should be made towards sealing any exposed cancellous surfaces with bone wax in

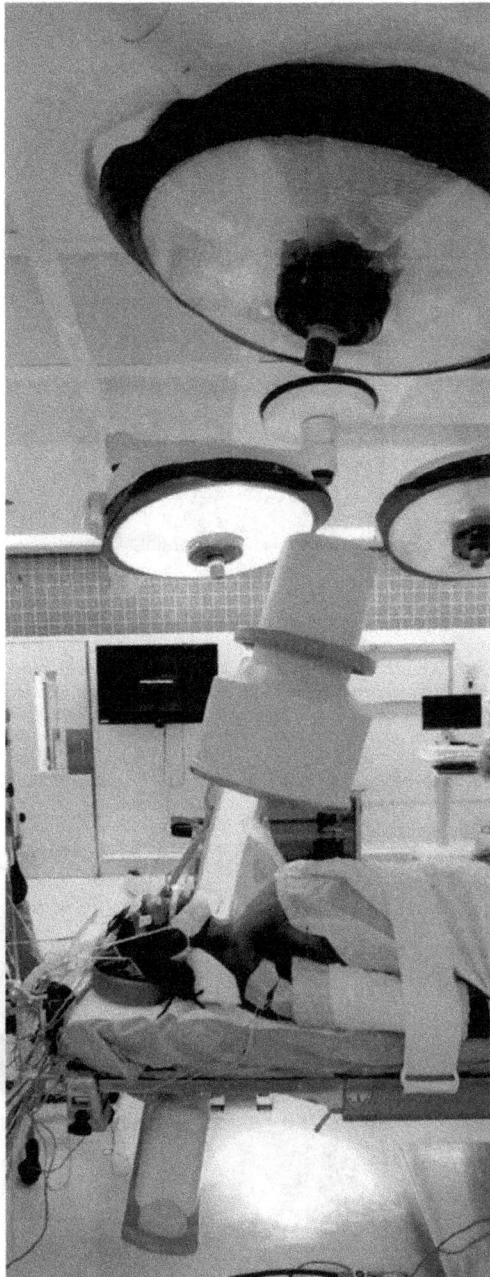

Figure 4.
Ferguson view is an AP view of the cervical disc space taken with opening of collimation and caudal tilt angulation of the x-ray tube 30° to 35°.

order to prevent heterotopic ossification. Next retractors can be repositioned at the adjacent level for placement of the fusion implant in standard fashion. If using a plate attention should be paid towards the proximity of the plate in regards to the adjacent disc space as this has be found to be the critical determinant of adjacent level heterotopic ossification [45, 46].

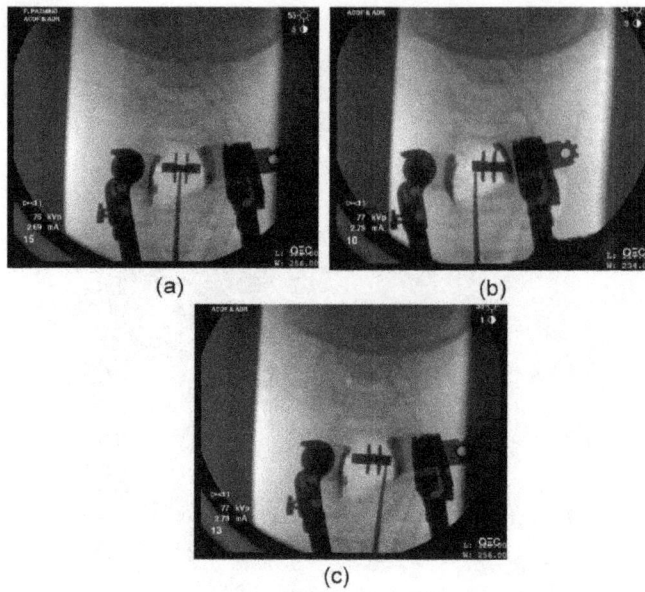

Figure 5.
(a) Proper midline positioning of the prosthesis can be confirmed fluoroscopically with placement of a nerve hook within the instrumentation until a center center "field goal" view is obtained. The nerve hook is clearly bisecting the flanges of the trial. Drilling in this orientation will lock in an appropriately midline positioned implant. (b) Improper midline placement: Here the nerve hook is no longer bisecting the flanges of the implant which confirms the implant is malrotated towards the right, the retractor needs to be loosened and repositioned so that the trial can be repositioned accordingly. (c) Improper midline placement: Here the nerve hook is no longer bisecting the flanges of the implant which confirms the implant is malrotated towards the left and needs to be repositioned accordingly.

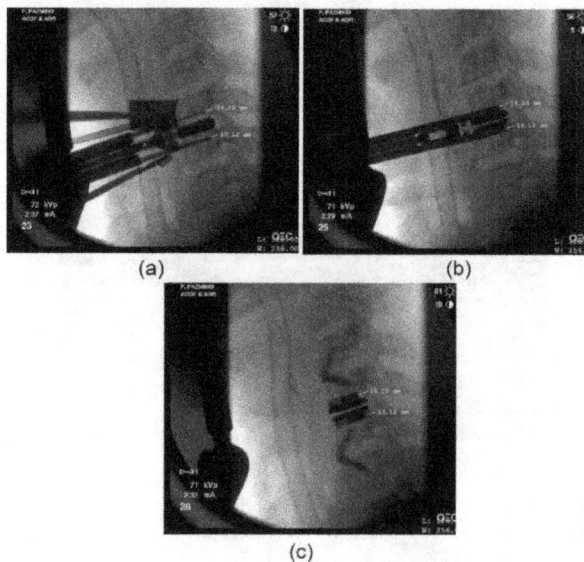

Figure 6.
(a) Prior to removal of the trial, discrete measurements can be taken to confirm the exact depth of the insertion of the drill bit. Measurements are obtained from the tip of the drill to the posterior margin of each vertebral body. (b) This depth can then be compared to the implant positioning as tapping occurs to confirm final placement of the arthroplasty. Measurements are obtained from the tip of the implant to the posterior margin of each vertebral body. (c) A final xray and measurements can be obtained to ensure the final implant has not moved after removal of the instrumentation. This will help confirm if any final tamping needs to be performed.

6. Case studies

6.1 Case 1 C56 ADR C67 ACDF

51 year old female who presents with cervical pains which she describes as 80% neck pain and 20% arm/shoulder pain, which is 100% left-sided in a C6 and C7 distribution. MRI of the cervical spine demonstrated a C5-C6 3 mm disc herniation with facet arthropathy and severe bilateral foraminal stenosis (**Figure 7a,b**). At C6-C7 a 2 mm left paracentral disc protrusion was noted with severe bilateral foraminal stenosis (**Figure 7c**). For her pain, the patient had tried a prolonged course of conservative management in the form of physical therapy, heating pads, and ice packs. She had tried medications in the form of NSAID's, muscle relaxants and narcotics. She had consulted with pain management and undergone injection procedures in the form of transforaminal epidural injections at C56 and later

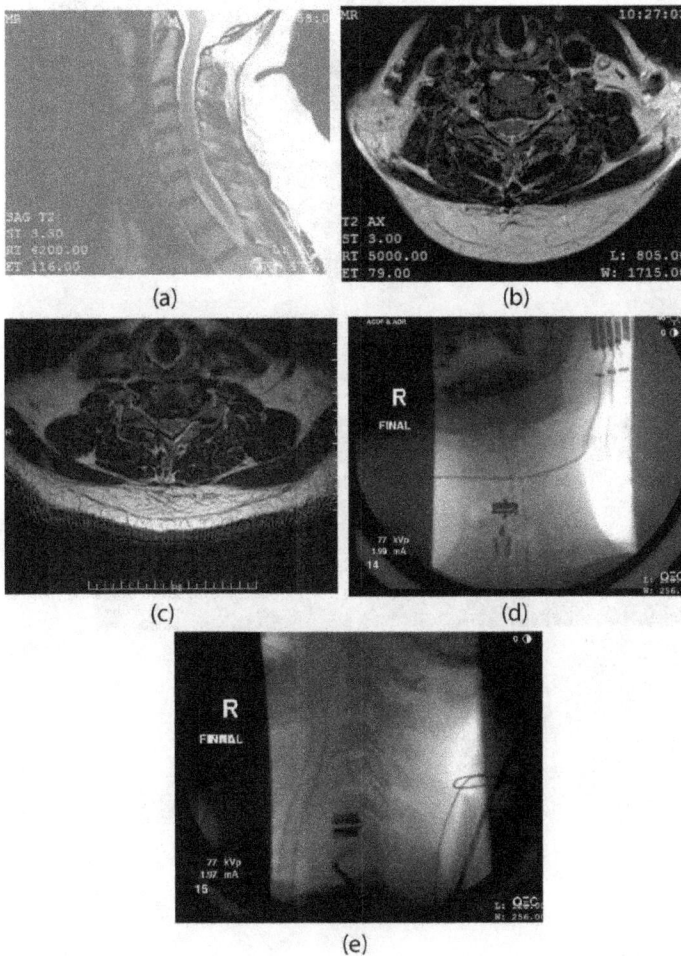

Figure 7.
(a) Sagittal MRI of the cervical spine demonstrated a C5-C6 and C67 disc herniations. (b) Axial MRI of the cervical spine demonstrated a C5-C6 bilobed herniation with severe bilateral foraminal stenosis. (c) At C6-C7 a 2 mm disc protrusion was noted with severe bilateral foraminal stenosis. (d) AP Xray artificial disc replacement at C56 and anterior cervical discectomy and fusion at C67. (e) Lateral Xray artificial disc replacement at C56 and anterior cervical discectomy and fusion at C67.

at C67, which each provided one hundred percent pain relief and lasted for one month. Patient underwent an uncomplicated Artificial Disc Replacement at C56 and Anterior Cervical Discectomy and Fusion at C67, and has since noted complete resolution of her symptoms (**Figure 7d, e**).

6.2 Case 2 C45 ACDF C56 ADR C67 ACDF

48 year-old female who presented with 95% neck pain and 5% shoulder pain, which is 50% right-sided and 50% left, sided in a C5, C6, and C7 distribution. MRI of the cervical spine demonstrated at the C4-C5 level moderate central spinal

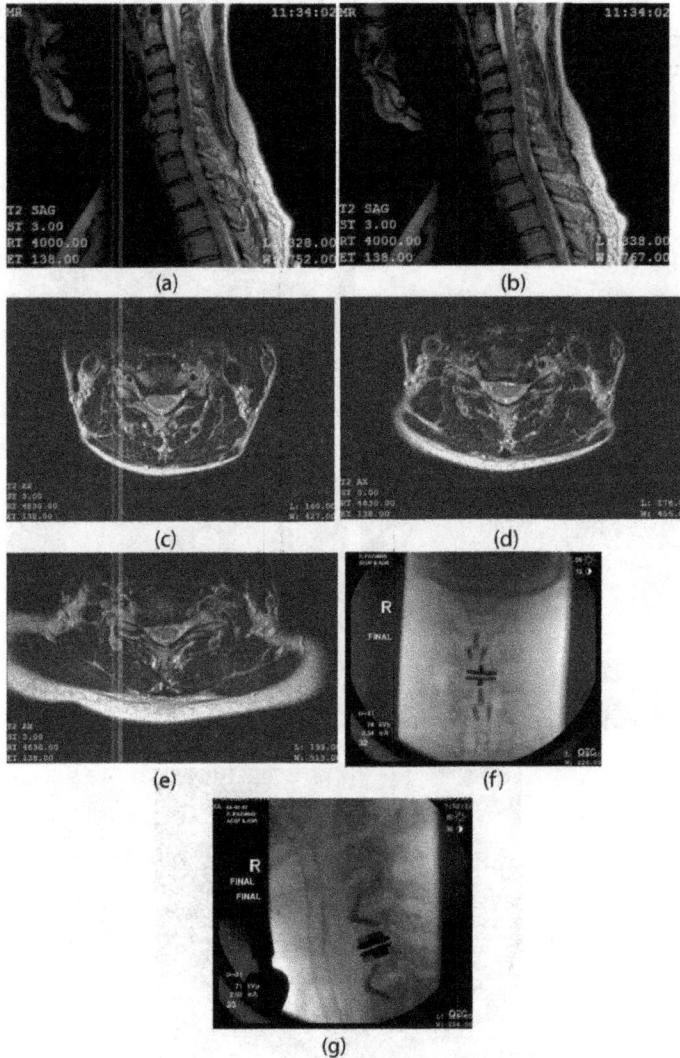

Figure 8.
(a, b) Sagittal MRI of the cervical spine demonstrated herniations at the C4-C5, C56, C67. (c) Axial MRI of the cervical spine demonstrated C45 large disc herniation with neuroforaminal stenosis. (d) Axial MRI of the cervical spine demonstrated 56 eccentric disc herniations with left sided neuroforaminal stenosis. (e) Axial MRI of the cervical spine demonstrated C67 eccentric disc herniation with right sided neuroforaminal stenosis. (f) AP Xray artificial disc replacement at C56 and anterior cervical discectomy and fusion at C45, and C67. (g) LATERAL Xray artificial disc replacement at C56 and anterior cervical discectomy and fusion at C45, and C67.

canal stenosis, a 4 mm disc protrusion with moderate-to-severe neural foraminal, narrowing bilaterally and impingement on the exiting nerve roots bilaterally **Figure 8a-c**. At the C5-C6, level, there was a 4 mm left paracentral disc protrusion with severe neural foraminal narrowing on the left and moderate foraminal narrowing on the right. There is impingement on the exiting nerve roots bilaterally greater on the left than the right (**Figure 8d**). At the C6-C7 level, there was a 5 mm right paracentral disc protrusion with severe neural foraminal narrowing on the right with impingement on the exiting nerve roots on the right (**Figure 8e**). There is moderate neural foraminal narrowing on the left and moderate central spinal canal stenosis. For her pain, the patient had tried a prolonged course of conservative management in the form of physical therapy, chiropractic treatment, heating pads, and ice packs. She had tried medications in the form of NSAID's, muscle relaxants and narcotics. She had consulted with pain management and undergone three injection procedures in the form of transforaminal epidural injections at C45, C56 and later at C67, each of which provided seventy percent pain relief and lasted for one to three months. Patient underwent an uncomplicated Artificial Disc Replacement at C56 and Anterior Cervical Discectomy and Fusion at C45 and C67, and has since noted resolution of her symptoms (**Figure 8f, g**).

7. Conclusions

In properly indicated patients, with meticulous preoperative planning and sound surgical technique, cervical hybrid arthroplasty offers an excellent surgical option and is a safe and effective alternative to multilevel fusion for the management of cervical radiculopathy and myelopathy.

Conflict of interest

"The authors declare no conflict of interest."

Author details

Pablo Pazmiño
SpineCal, Santa Monica, CA, USA

*Address all correspondence to: doctor@spinecal.com

IntechOpen

References

[1] Kim Y-S, Park J-Y, Moon BJ, Kim S-D, Lee J-K. Is stand alone PEEK cage the gold standard in multilevel anterior cervical discectomy and fusion (ACDF)? Results of a minimum 1-year follow up. J Clin Neurosci. 2018 Jan;47:341-346.

[2] Flynn TB. Neurologic Complications of Anterior Cervical Interbody Fusion [Internet]. Vol. 7, Spine. 1982. p. 536-9. Available from: http://dx.doi.org/10.1097/00007632-198211000-00004

[3] Barysh O, Fedoryna E. COMPLICATIONS AND MISTAKES AFTER ANTERIOR CERVICAL INTERBODY FUSION WITH AUTOLOGOUS BONE GRAFTS [Internet]. Vol. 0, ORTHOPAEDICS, TRAUMATOLOGY and PROSTHETICS. 2014. p. 97. Available from: http://dx.doi.org/10.15674/0030-59872014497-103

[4] Qian B. P100. Analysis of failure and complications associated with anterior cervical fusion cage [Internet]. Vol. 4, The Spine Journal. 2004. p. S112. Available from: http://dx.doi.org/10.1016/j.spinee.2004.05.228

[5] Murrey D, Janssen M, Delamarter R, Goldstein J, Zigler J, Tay B, et al. 152. 5-Year Results of the Prospective, Randomized, Multicenter FDA Investigational Device Exemption (IDE) ProDisc-C TDR Clinical Trial [Internet]. Vol. 9, The Spine Journal. 2009. p. 80S. Available from: http://dx.doi.org/10.1016/j.spinee.2009.08.188

[6] Murrey D, Janssen M, Delamarter R, Goldstein J, Zigler J, Tay B, et al. Results of the prospective, randomized, controlled multicenter Food and Drug Administration investigational device exemption study of the ProDisc-C total disc replacement versus anterior discectomy and fusion for the treatment

of 1-level symptomatic cervical disc disease. Spine J. 2009 Apr;9(4):275-286.

[7] Delamarter R, Zigler JE, Balderston RA, Cammisa FP, Goldstein JA, Spivak JM. Prospective, randomized, multicenter Food and Drug Administration investigational device exemption study of the ProDisc-L Total Disc Replacement compared with circumferential arthrodesis for the treatment of two-level lumbar degenerative disc disease: results at twenty-four monthsJ Bone Joint Surg Am 2011;93(8):705-15. Epub 2011 Mar 11 [Internet]. Vol. 11, The Spine Journal. 2011. p. 793. Available from: http://dx.doi.org/10.1016/j.spinee.2011.08.423

[8] Zigler JE, Delamarter RB. Five-year results of the prospective, randomized, multicenter, Food and Drug Administration investigational device exemption study of the ProDisc-L total disc replacement versus circumferential arthrodesis for the treatment of single-level degenerative disc disease [Internet]. Vol. 17, Journal of Neurosurgery: Spine. 2012. p. 493-501. Available from: http://dx.doi.org/10.3171/2012.9.spine11498

[9] Kearns S, Janssen M, Murrey D, Delamarter R. Five-Year Results of the Prodisc-C Multicenter Randomized Clinical Trial [Internet]. Vol. 11, The Spine Journal. 2011. p. S46. Available from: http://dx.doi.org/10.1016/j.spinee.2011.08.120

[10] Murrey DB, Zigler JE, Delamarter RB, Spivak JM, Janssen ME. Seven-Year Results of the ProDisc-C Multicenter Randomized Clinical Trial [Internet]. Vol. 12, The Spine Journal. 2012. p. S61-2. Available from: http://dx.doi.org/10.1016/j.spinee.2012.08.181

[11] Anderson PA, Nassr A, Currier BL, Sebastian AS, Arnold PM, Fehlings MG,

et al. Evaluation of Adverse Events in Total Disc Replacement: A Meta-Analysis of FDA Summary of Safety and Effectiveness Data. Global Spine J. 2017 Apr;7(1 Suppl):76S – 83S.

[12] Hollyer MA, Gill EC, Ayis S, Demetriades AK. The safety and efficacy of hybrid surgery for multilevel cervical degenerative disc disease versus anterior cervical discectomy and fusion or cervical disc arthroplasty: a systematic review and meta-analysis. Acta Neurochir. 2020 Feb;162(2):289-303.

[13] He J, Ding C, Liu H, Wu T, Huang K, Hong Y, et al. Does Fusion Affect Anterior Bone Loss in Adjacent Cervical Disc Arthroplasty in Contiguous Two-Level Hybrid Surgery? World Neurosurg. 2020 Nov;143:e127–e135.

[14] Boddapati V, Lee NJ, Mathew J, Vulapalli MM, Lombardi JM, Dyrszka MD, et al. Hybrid Anterior Cervical Discectomy and Fusion and Cervical Disc Arthroplasty: An Analysis of Short-Term Complications, Reoperations, and Readmissions. Global Spine J. 2020 Jul 24;2192568220941453.

[15] Cardoso MJ, Mendelsohn A, Rosner MK. Cervical hybrid arthroplasty with 2 unique fusion techniques. J Neurosurg Spine. 2011 Jul;15(1):48-54.

[16] Mehren C, Wuertz-Kozak K, Sauer D, Hitzl W, Pehlivanoglu T, Heider F. Implant Design and the Anchoring Mechanism Influence the Incidence of Heterotopic Ossification in Cervical Total Disc Replacement at 2-year Follow-up. Spine. 2019 Nov 1;44(21):1471-1480.

[17] Zeng J, Liu H, Chen H, Ding C, Rong X, Meng Y, et al. Comparison of Heterotopic Ossification After Fixed- and Mobile-Core Cervical Disc Arthroplasty. World Neurosurg. 2018 Dec;120:e1319–e1324.

[18] Hamby WB, Glaser HT. Replacement of spinal intervertebral discs with locally polymerizing methyl methacrylate: experimental study of effects upon tissues and report of a small clinical series. J Neurosurg. 1959 May;16(3):311-313.

[19] Cleveland DA. The use of methylacrylic for spinal stabilization after disc operations. Marquette Med Rev. 1955;20:62-64.

[20] FASSIO, B. Discal prosthesis made of silicone : experimental study and 1st clinical cases. Nouv Presse Med. 1978;7:207.

[21] Cummins BH, Robertson JT, Gill SS. Surgical experience with an implanted artificial cervical joint. J Neurosurg. 1998 Jun;88(6):943-948.

[22] Hui N, Phan K, Kerferd J, Lee M, Mobbs RJ. Comparison of M6-C and Mobi-C cervical total disc replacement for cervical degenerative disc disease in adults. J Spine Surg. 2019 Dec;5(4):393-403.

[23] Mehren C, Heider F, Sauer D, Kothe R, Korge A, Hitzl W, et al. Clinical and Radiological Outcome of a New Total Cervical Disc Replacement Design. Spine. 2019 Feb 15;44(4):E202–E210.

[24] Markwalder T-M, Wenger M, Marbacher S. A 6.5-year follow-up of 14 patients who underwent ProDisc total disc arthroplasty for combined long-standing degenerative lumbar disc disease and recent disc herniation [Internet]. Vol. 18, Journal of Clinical Neuroscience. 2011. p. 1677-81. Available from: http://dx.doi.org/10.1016/j.jocn.2011.04.024

[25] Pitsika M, Nissen J. Spinal cord compression due to nucleus migration from Mobi-C total disc replacement [Internet]. British Journal of Neurosurgery. 2020. p. 1-4. Available

from: http://dx.doi.org/10.1080/026886
97.2020.1716942

[26] Byval'tsev VA, Kalinin AA,
Stepanov IA, Pestryakov YY,
Shepelev VV. [Analysis of the results of
total cervical disc arthroplasty using a
M6-C prosthesis: a multicenter study].
Zh Vopr Neirokhir Im N N Burdenko.
2017;81(5):46-55.

[27] McAfee PC. Classification of
Heterotopic Ossification in Artificial
Disc Replacement [Internet]. The
Artificial Disc. 2003. p. 157-163.
Available from: http://dx.doi.
org/10.1007/978-3-662-05347-8_14

[28] Harris L, Dyson E, Elliot M,
Peterson D, Ulbricht C, Casey A.
Delayed periprosthetic collection after
cervical disc arthroplasty. J Neurosurg
Spine. 2019 Dec 13;1-8.

[29] Lind B, Sihlbom H, Nordwall A,
Malchau H. Normal range of motion
of the cervical spine. Arch Phys Med
Rehabil. 1989 Sep;70(9):692-695.

[30] Panjabi MM, Duranceau J,
Goel V, Oxland T, Takata K. Cervical
human vertebrae. Quantitative
three-dimensional anatomy of the
middle and lower regions. Spine. 1991
Aug;16(8):861-869.

[31] White AA, Panjabi MM. Clinical
Biomechanics of the Spine. Lippincott
Williams & Wilkins; 1978. 534 p.

[32] Panjabi MM, Ito S, Pearson AM,
Ivancic PC. Injury Mechanisms of the
Cervical Intervertebral Disc During
Simulated Whiplash [Internet]. Vol. 29,
Spine. 2004. p. 1217-25. Available from:
http://dx.doi.org/10.1097/00007632-
200406010-00011

[33] White AA, Panjabi MM.
Biomechanical Considerations
in the Surgical Management of
Cervical Spondylotic Myelopathy
[Internet]. Vol. 13, Spine. 1988. p.

856-60. Available from: http://dx.doi.
org/10.1097/00007632-198807000-
00029

[34] Buchowski JM, Daniel Riew K.
Primary Indications and Disc
Space Preparation for Cervical
Disc Arthroplasty [Internet].
Motion Preservation Surgery of the
Spine. 2008. p. 185-192. Available
from: http://dx.doi.org/10.1016/
b978-1-4160-3994-5.10021-3

[35] Wu T-K, Meng Y, Wang B-Y, Hong Y,
Rong X, Ding C, et al. Is the behavior
of disc replacement adjacent to fusion
affected by the location of the fused
level in hybrid surgery? [Internet].
Vol. 18, The Spine Journal. 2018. p.
2171-80. Available from: http://dx.doi.
org/10.1016/j.spinee.2018.04.019

[36] Wu T-K, Meng Y, Liu H, Wang B-Y,
Hong Y, Rong X, et al. Biomechanical
effects on the intermediate segment
of noncontiguous hybrid surgery with
cervical disc arthroplasty and anterior
cervical discectomy and fusion: a
finite element analysis [Internet].
Vol. 19, The Spine Journal. 2019. p.
1254-63. Available from: http://dx.doi.
org/10.1016/j.spinee.2019.02.004

[37] Hu L, Wu T, Liu H, Wang B,
Zhang J, Meng Y, et al. Influence of
Fusion on the Behavior of Adjacent Disc
Arthroplasty in Contiguous 2-Level
Hybrid Surgery In Vivo [Internet].
Vol. 132, World Neurosurgery. 2019. p.
e929-40. Available from: http://dx.doi.
org/10.1016/j.wneu.2019.07.073

[38] Wu T-K, Meng Y, Liu H, Hong Y,
Wang B-Y, Rong X, et al. Primary
cervical disc arthroplasty versus
cervical disc arthroplasty adjacent to
previous fusion [Internet]. Vol. 97,
Medicine. 2018. p. e11755. Available
from: http://dx.doi.org/10.1097/
md.0000000000011755

[39] Park DK, Lin EL, Phillips FM. Index
and Adjacent Level Kinematics After

Cervical Disc Replacement and Anterior Fusion [Internet]. Vol. 36, Spine. 2011. p. 721-30. Available from: http://dx.doi.org/10.1097/brs.0b013e3181df10fc

[40] Hyun Y-S, Park J-S, Song K-W, Kim G-L, Lee J-Y, Shin J-H. Clinical and Radiographic Results of Artificial Disc Replacement Combined with Anterior Cervical Discectomy and Fusion Versus Two-Level Anterior Cervical Discectomy and Fusion in Two-Level Cervical Disc Disease [Internet]. Vol. 24, Journal of Korean Society of Spine Surgery. 2017. p. 211. Available from: http://dx.doi.org/10.4184/jkss.2017.24.4.211

[41] Meng Y, Wang X, Zhao Z, Wang B, Wu T, Liu H. Intraoperative Anterior Migration of the Prestige-LP Cervical Disc Owing to an Inappropriate Implantation Sequence During Continuous 2-Level Artificial Cervical Disc Replacement: A Case Report with 8-Year Follow-Up [Internet]. Vol. 116, World Neurosurgery. 2018. p. 194-200. Available from: http://dx.doi.org/10.1016/j.wneu.2018.05.093

[42] Chen J, Wang X, Yuan W, Tang Y, Zhang Y, Wan M. Cervical myelopathy after cervical total disc arthroplasty: case report and literature review. Spine. 2012 May 1;37(10):E624–E628.

[43] Wang X-F, Meng Y, Liu H, Hong Y, Wang B-Y. Surgical strategy used in multilevel cervical disc replacement and cervical hybrid surgery: Four case reports. World J Clin Cases. 2020 Sep 6;8(17):3890-3902.

[44] Patel VV, Andrews C, Pradhan BB, Bae HW, Kanim LEA, Kropf MA, et al. Computed tomography assessment of the accuracy of in vivo placement of artificial discs in the lumbar spine including radiographic and clinical consequences. Spine. 2006 Apr 15;31(8):948-953.

[45] Li L. Re: Yang JY, Song HS, Lee M, et al. Adjacent level ossification

development after anterior cervical fusion without plate fixation. Spine 2009;34:30-3. Spine. 2009 Jul 1;34(15):1626-1627; author reply 1627.

[46] Yang J-Y, Song H-S, Lee M, Bohlman HH, Riew KD. Adjacent level ossification development after anterior cervical fusion without plate fixation. Spine. 2009 Jan 1;34(1):30-33.

Chapter 3

Cervical Arthroplasty

Jason M. Highsmith

Abstract

Technological advances have allowed spine surgery to follow the trend toward minimally invasive surgery in general. Specifically, we have seen a corresponding rise in the popularity of cervical arthroplasty. For the treatment of cervical disc disease, arthroplasty is a less invasive option than the gold standard of cervical discectomy and arthrodesis, which by nature is more disruptive to surrounding tissues. Arthroplasty preserves the facets, maintains motion, and reduces the rate of adjacent segment breakdown. These factors counteract the negative impacts of fusion while maintaining the benefits. Arthroplasty implants themselves have become more streamlined to implant as well with less native bone destruction, and biomechanics more compatible with the native disc. While initial implants were ball and socket devices with complex fixation and plane-specific movements, later devices incorporated such motions as translation and compression. Viscoelastic components and materials more closely resembling native tissues afford a more biocompatible implant profile. Until cell-based therapies can successfully reproduce native tissue, we will rely on artificial components that closely resemble and assimilate them.

Keywords: cervical disc replacement, arthroplasty, cervical fusion, artificial disc, implants

1. Introduction

In the trend toward minimally invasive surgery, operations for the cervical spine have followed a similar tendency. While microsurgery has been in the lexicon of neurosurgery for ages, one of the earliest uses of the term "minimally invasive" in spine surgery was used by Probst in 1989 to discuss lumbar microdiscectomy [1]. While the term "minimally invasive" has become somewhat of a generic moniker for many different approaches, its intent is to be less traumatic to the patient with lower complication rates.

In the cervical spine, midline sparing posterior procedures such as lateral [2] and far later posterior approaches have afforded the opportunity to use smaller incisions and even endoscopic [3] approaches. Anterior foraminotomy, a disc preserving approach, has also been proposed [4] with favorable results [5]. However, these approaches have given limited access to midline pathologies and offer little benefit for cases with central herniation or instability.

Anterior discectomy alone allows central pathology to be addressed with reasonable success but high reoperation rates [6]. The addition of fusion stabilizes the spine in addition to maintaining distraction and neural foramen patency. Interbody grafts were instrumental in providing this indirect decompression and additional stability. Fusion halts further disc degeneration, preserves sagittal balance, and eliminates segmental instability. Cervical fusion surgery, particularly anterior approaches has followed this minimally invasive trend and become more streamlined.

The anterior cervical discectomy and fusion (ACDF) was first reported in 1955 by Robinson and Smith [7], and this approach quickly became the dominant approach. While the competing Cloward technique [8] offered a high cancellous surface area for fusion, it had a high rate of graft collapse [9] and subsidence rates of up to 9.6% [10]. The shape of the graft provides some intrinsic stability but endplate preparation is more invasive requiring significantly more native bone removal which also predisposed patients to kyphosis [9, 11] at rates up to 9.6% [10]. Furthermore, higher complication rates include up to 4.8% of neurologic injuries [10].

The Smith-Robinson technique [12] is less invasive given that it is endplate sparing and causes minimal vertebral body destruction. It also provides better visualization of the decompression, particularly the uncovertebral joints. Arthrodesis by either technique has proven an effective treatment for cervical spondylosis and disc herniation [9, 13–15]. Anterior discectomy with fusion has been the prominent surgical treatment for symptomatic cervical spondylosis for over 60 years. Traditionally, bone dowels or spacers were harvested from autologous iliac crest contributing to hip pain rates of up to 39% [16]. This additional procedure has contributed to the relatively longer hospital stays of ACDF patients [17].

Allograft iliac crest provided a respite from further surgical trauma at a second site and was thus less invasive. However, fashioning an appropriate size graft added additional operating time on the back table. Pre-cut fibular strut grafts offered a more convenient and efficient option but are limited in terms of footprint size and have a high cortical to cancellous bone concentration. Machined structural allograft was the next iteration providing greater surface area of the graft and a higher percentage of cancellous bone contact, albeit at a greater cost.

Nonunion and graft subsidence still occurred and titanium plating developed as a more stable option [18]. The plate and four screw construct provided a solid fixation for arthrodesis to occur. With fusion rates of up to 100% [19], this technique became the gold standard for 20+ years. While the uniplate had some early adopters [20], high pseudofusion rates were reported [21].

With load-bearing limitations, limited allograft supply, and concerns over disease transmission from cadaveric bone, titanium cages had a simultaneous rise in popularity particularly in the lumbar spine. The imaging artifact and subsidence of titanium as well as its limited machining options increased the demand for synthetic polymers such as poly ether ether ketone (PEEK). In the cervical spine particularly, PEEK offered the ability to have a number of footprint options as well as height options for corpectomy and multilevel constructs.

The latest stage of cervical fusion has allowed titanium mini plates to incorporate with PEEK spacers as a stand-alone option with internal fixation (**Figure 1**). This integral plate allows for less bony exposure and potentially less issues with longus colli bleeding, recurrent laryngeal paresis, and sympathetic chain injury at lower levels. Furthermore, the zero- or low-profile interbody plate, as opposed to an on-lay plate, has been shown to have shorter surgical times and lower rates of dysphagia [22]. In addition, these implants have been shown to have lower rates of adjacent segment degeneration (ASD) [23–25]. However, these implants have been associated with increased rates of kyphosis [26, 27].

While the technological advances in arthrodesis have given rise to faster procedures and shorter stays, there has been a concordant rise in cost from zero-dollar autograft to modern-day single-level constructs costing $5–6 K a level. At a time when physician reimbursement is diminishing this rise in per case cost is concerning, although the cost–benefit may be worth it for reduced surgeon's time.

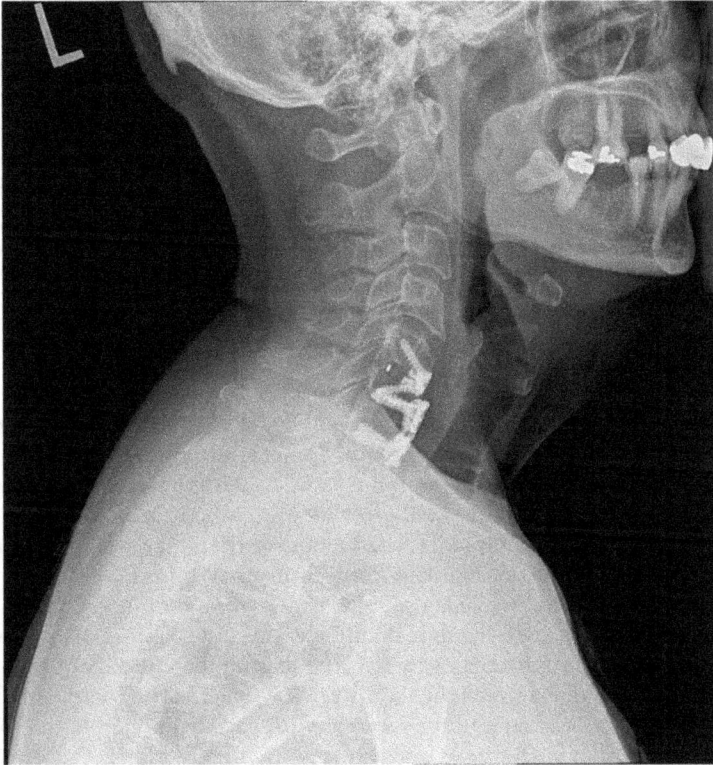

Figure 1.
Cervical fusion devices showing zero-profile devicie at C5–6 and standard allograft and four screw plate at C6–7.

2. Problems with fusion

Cervical fusion is known to alter spinal biomechanics by creating abnormal loads and affecting segmental motion at adjacent vertebrae [28, 29]. These changes may accelerate adjacent disc degeneration through the increased stress on the adjacent disc [29–31].

Multiple studies have documented evidence of adjacent segment level disease including radiographic findings of new anterior osteophyte formation or enlargement, increased narrowing of an interspace, new DDD, and calcification of the anterior longitudinal ligament [31]. Fusion has shown an increased rate of these compared to arthroplasty. Similarly, the rate of symptomatic disease along with the need for medical treatments related to such was also greater in the fusion cohort.

Multilevel fusion constructs demonstrate even greater stress [32]. These multi-level procedures had higher rates of reoperation, pseudoarthrosis, and complications [33, 34] compared to single-level constructs.

3. The case for arthroplasty

While the ACDF has been the gold standard for years, the well-known effects of motion loss and adjacent segment breakdown have been driving factors for cervical arthroplasty. One such mechanism is the neighboring intradiscal pressure. Fusion constructs produce greater neighboring intradiscal pressure [30] compared to arthroplasty which preserves physiologic intradiscal pressures at neighboring levels.

In essence, arthroplasty is itself less invasive than fusion because of maintained motion and reducing the need for adjacent level surgery. Like the ACDF, cervical arthroplasty has followed a similar trend toward less invasiveness with a more streamlined process and less procedural time. The nomenclature for this procedure has varied markedly to include: anterior cervical discectomy and arthroplasty (ACDA, and abbreviated ACA), artificial disc replacement (ADR), total disc replacement (TDR), cervical total disc replacement (cTDR), cervical disc replacement (CDR), and cervical disc arthroplasty (CDA).

4. Design rationale

An arthroplasty device must replicate the native disc as much as possible. Three primary considerations include: maintaining intervertebral spacing, allowing for motion with the segment, and maintaining stability with the bones neighboring the segment. The initial stability with screw fixation was the primary focus of early implants while more recent implants relied on press-fit, teeth, and/or keels as well as ligamentum taxis for initial stability. Long-term stability involves ingrowth of bone into porous endplates while at the same time allowing for revision.

The placement of an artificial disc should be done with limited disruption of surrounding anatomy. Arthroplasty by nature relies on the integrity of the neighboring facet joints and ligaments for stability. Likewise, the functioning arthroplasty device should not overload the facets nor unload them.

Replicating motion in all planes but also constraining motion means the device has to mirror physiologic tissue in terms of biomechanics. In addition to allowing loading, flexion/extension, rotation, and lateral bending, the arthroplasty device should optimally allow for translation as well (**Figure 2**). Ideally, the device would have some natural shock absorption for axial forces. This proved to be a limiting factor in early devices but more modern devices have incorporated this.

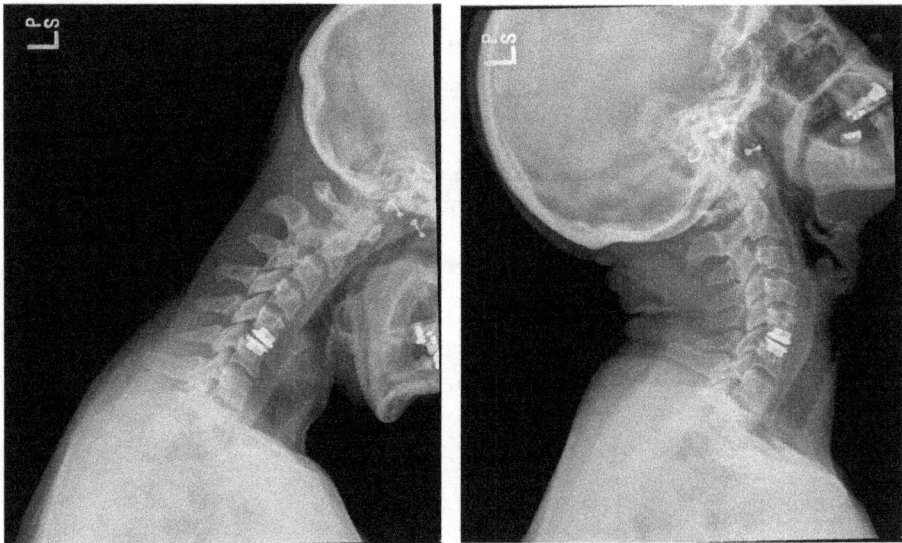

Figure 2.
Flexion/extension views of the Centinel spine ProDisc-C at C5–6 show arthroplasty device flexing and extending with the spine.

The movement within the implant must be balanced by a stable bone-implant interface anchoring the implant. While a fusion allows for the remodeling of bone, arthroplasty is not afforded such long-term stability. The endplates must allow for a proper degree of bony on-growth while maintaining physiologic loads at this interface to reduce implant failure and endplate failure. The resilience of the implant over the patient's life span is also an important factor. In the event of implant failure, the design should allow for minimal impact from this failure and ideally offer a radiographic cue to its existence.

Implant material is another factor that must be considered in normal usage. Materials should be chosen that are biocompatible, durable, minimize wear debris, and have a minimal inflammatory response. Additionally, materials should be selected that minimize diagnostic imaging artifact at the index level, but certainly preserving visualization of the adjacent segments is essential.

5. History of arthroplasty

While fusion has been the gold standard for over sixty years, arthroplasty designs have been developing over a similar time frame. Dr. Ulf Fernstrom studied a spherical intercorporeal endoprosthesis, or simply a stainless-steel ball, placed in the disc space in the late 1950s. He implanted 191 of his "Fernstrom Balls" in the cervical and lumbar spines of 101 patients [35]. The procedure was later abandoned over high failure rates with subsidence, migration, and hypermobility. Methylmethacrylate [36] was used as an alternative to the steel ball but did not gain much traction in the spine world.

Arthroplasty progress was somewhat dormant for approximately 30 years until the stainless-steel ball and socket implants from Bristol/Cummins were developed [37]. These advanced into a ball and trough design that allowed for translational movement to become the commercially available Prestige line from Medtronic. Charite was approved in 2004 as the first FDA-approved commercial spinal arthroplasty device (lumbar spine). Prestige ST was approved in 2007 as the first cervical arthroplasty device. This steel on steel implant was simple but its stainless-steel construction caused significant artifact on MR imaging. Some patients reported clicking sounds from the saddle joint (personal experience). The esthetics and dysphagia of an on-lay plate (Prestige-ST) as well as time-consuming implant procedure with four screw fixation.

Prestige LP was first marketed OUS in 2004 and approved by FDA in 2014. It was a less invasive approach in terms of fixation. As named, the LP design relied on lower-profile press-fit rales and antimigration teeth for fixation. It also had a titanium plasma spray for additional fixation. The implant was also made with a titanium ceramic composite material that provided better imaging characteristics. Arthroplasty implants designed up to this point allowed motion but no elasticity. The elasticity component is key for load-damping properties.

Early arthroplasty devices like the Bristol and Prestige-ST had a prominent four screw construct with a locking mechanism. Subsequent revisions like the Prestige-LP had a lower profile as so named along with no need for screw fixation.

Similar to the trends toward less invasive, more modern implants have also followed the trend toward more physiologic motion. Early arthroplasty devices mirrored general orthopedic implants with two articulating surfaces. In this spine, these first-generation implants relied on metal articulations attached to the endplate above and below the index disc (Bristol and Prestige). The early Bristol disc was a ball and socket which allows lateral bending, rotation, and flexion/extension but not translation. Prestige was created with a trough on the lower articulating surface in order to allow anterior/posterior translation.

General orthopedic implants evolved to incorporate a plastic spacer in hopes of reducing metallic wear debris while also providing better wear characteristics and a minor degree of shock absorption. A high molecular weight polyethylene core was juxtaposed between the metal surfaces. These second-generation devices reduced some of the metal-on-metal concerns but still lacked elasticity like a native disc. The ProDisc returned to a ball and socket approach with the bottom half of the polyethylene core anchored to the inferior endplate. The subsequently released Secure-C preserved the superior ball and socket design but had a saddle design on the inferior endplate articulating surface. This allowed for translation.

6. Arthroplasty 2.0

The first generation of arthroplasty implants replicated conventional orthopedic implants with metal-on-metal articulating surfaces. These types of implants allow rotation, lateral bending, flexion and extension, and in some cases (Prestige-ST) anterolisthesis.

Implants with a polyethylene core have offered more physiologic movement and less concern over metallic deposition and blood levels. These second-generation implants like ProDisc offered a fixed core while the subsequently released Secure-C offered a sliding arthrodesis.

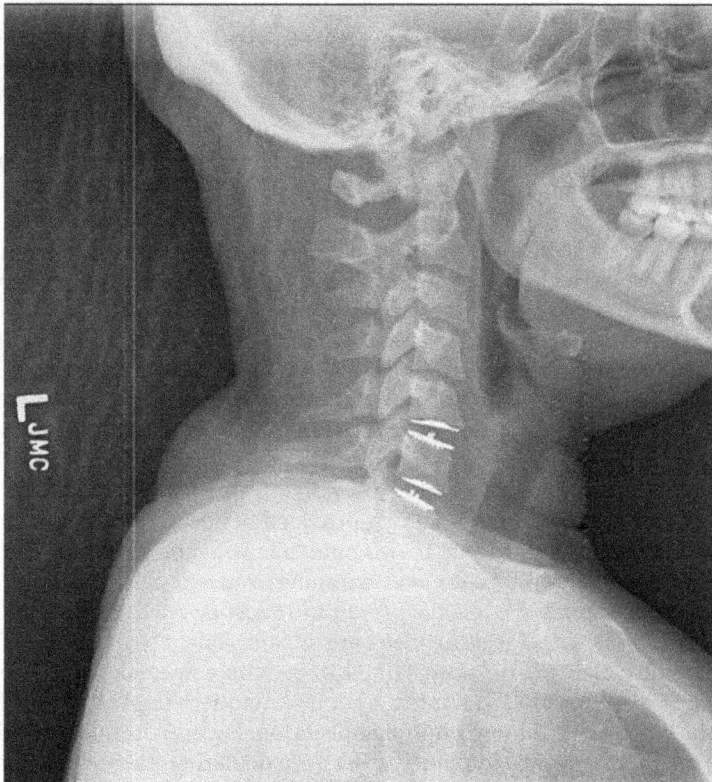

Figure 3.
The Zimmer Mobi-C was the first arthroplasty device to gain FDA approval in the United States for two-level indications.

Keel base implants like the ProDisc and Secure-C had no additional fixation hardware relaying on press-fit, bony on-growth, and keel anchoring stability. Even within the keel-based implants, the Secure-C introduced a shorter, wider keel which required even less exposure in a cranial-caudal direction.

The Nuvasive PCM disc allowed similar translation while also incorporating an arrow-shaped row of teeth as the primary fixation modality. When Mobi-C was released, the mindset was to perform as little endplate preparation as needed. Mobi-C went a step further to offer a circumferentially mobile center of rotation and obtained FDA approval as a two-level implant in 2013 (**Figure 3**).

While Mobi-C provided even more range of motion, concerns arose regarding hypermobility [38, 39] of the joint and the inability to adequately visualize the mobile core. With a mobile core, there was now a superior and inferior articulating surface to be concerned with, especially in sheer force loading.

7. Arthroplasty 3.0

Third-generation implants have allowed for translation and compression forces that more closely resemble physiologic motion.

The Bryan cervical disc was under development as early as 1997 by Spinal Dynamics Corporation. This implant relied on the preservation of the natural vertebral concavities with convex titanium shells matching them. The convex portion of the implant has a rough porous coating for bony on-growth. The concave surface of the implant is surrounded by a flexible membrane and lubricant to reduce friction and prevent migration of wear debris. The inner polymer nucleus provides a full range of motion while also allowing for a full range of motion but without loading. The Bryan disc eliminated the need for chiseling of keels but required a complex endplate preparation rig and procedure to shape the vertebral endplates. Subsequent implants like M6 likewise require only a small amount of chiseling for stability.

The Orthotic M6 implant has additional design components that allow more physiologic motions and replicate the physiological phenomenon of progressive resistance to motion in all six degrees of freedom (**Figure 4**). This design enables the disc to move in all six degrees, with independent angular rotations (flexion-extension, lateral bending, and axial rotation) along with independent translational motions (anterior–posterior and medial-lateral translations), as well as axial compression. This unique compressive ability has been thought to reduce adjacent segment disease specifically.

The M6 is a complex, multi-component implant that contains an artificial nucleus made of Viscoelastic polymer (PCU) designed to simulate the native nucleus structure. It lies adjacent to but is not fixated to two inner titanium endplates. This core nucleus is retained circumferentially between the titanium endplates by a fiber annulus matrix.

This Ultra High Molecular Weight Polyethylene (UHMWPE) fiber matrix is designed to simulate the native annular structure and is wound in a specific pattern, with multiple redundant layers. The matrix is wound around the core and through slots in the two Ti6Al4V titanium alloy inner endplates. Surrounding the flexible portions of the implant is a jacket of viscoelastic polymer (PCU) designed to minimize tissue in-growth and debris migration.

The inner plates are welded to outer plates the surface of which includes low profile fins and are coated with titanium plasma spray (TPS).

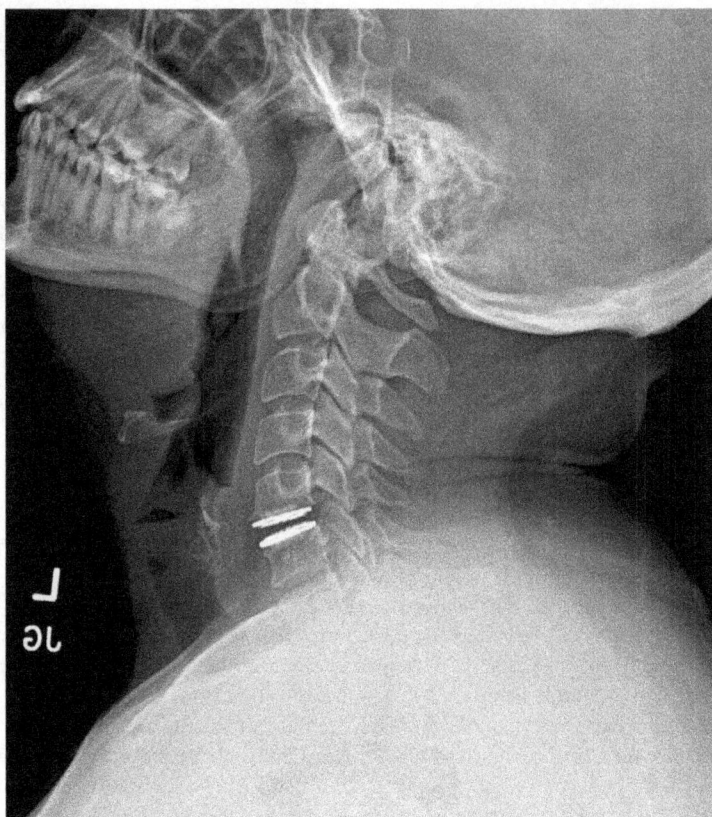

Figure 4.
The Orthofix M-6 implant allows for compressive axial loading.

8. Arthroplasty benefits

Numerous IDE studies have shown the benefits of arthroplasty over fusion, particularly in the cervical spine. In addition to being motion sparing, arthroplasty's perhaps greater value is in the reduction of adjacent segment breakdown. Several studies have shown lower rates of ASD in patients having undergone arthroplasty compared to their ACDF cohorts. The Secure-C study showed a 4x greater risk of having adjacent segment surgery in the ACDF group.

Lower rates of adjacent segment surgery, not only benefit patients could lower total health care costs. Ironically, this advantage has not been a motivating factor in insurance approval. The author spoke with the Medical Director of one major health insurance provider extolling the benefits of arthroplasty for a 24-year-old patient for whom a single-level ACDF was already approved. In an attempt to get authorization for an artificial disc at C5–6, I said, "I am fighting to get paid less for an operation that will potentially save the patient another surgery and in the end save you money on all accounts." Their response was, "We don't care. Our data shows most patients will change insurance carriers in the next five or six years and that doesn't help us." (Jason Highsmith, personal communication January 2009.)

Another potential benefit of this reduction of ASD is the ability to only operate on a symptomatic or freshly herniated level and leave other levels with some pathology untreated. In the past, there was a tendency to fuse everything that was abnormal, which of course exacerbates adjacent segment breakdown. This single-level approach for arthroplasty may lead to lower future costs.

ACDF patients had a higher reoperation rate at the index level in most of the IDE studies. Patients underwent a revision for nonunion as well as hardware revisions for screw pullout and plate fracture. One possible explanation is that most surgeons in the IDE study were highly skilled with ACDF procedures and took more time with the ACA procedure with better carpentry and decompression.

One explanation for this is that with arthroplasty there is only one active surface the articulating surface, whereas in ACDF there are two active surfaces of fusion to account for. Because of the need for additional decompression and resection of the uncovertebral joint, more care may be taken during ACA procedures.

Another positive factor for arthroplasty is certainly patient demand and satisfaction. The nomenclature of fusion is rarely a welcome term in clinical practice. At the same time, some patients with significant facet arthropathy or spondyloarthropathy come wanting disc replacement as the latest innovation regardless of their underlying pathology.

One limitation of the early studies was that the control group consisted of allograft spacers with a four-screw on-lay construct. While this was no doubt standard of care at the time these studies were initiated, and potentially still is, new options exist. Stand-alone devices with a cage and integrated plating are an easier construct to implant than a four screw on-lay plates.

While the clinical inclusion criteria for arthroplasty have been fairly stable over the last 20 years, the trend clinically has been more aggressive in indications. Initially, the ideal candidate was a less than 40-year-old patient with a solitary fresh disc, minimal adjacent segment disease, and little spondylosis. Now we are seeing older patients with more chronic disc issues, absent of facet pathology, undergoing arthroplasty. Based on my experience as a principal investigator for three IDE studies, we are seeing arthroplasty being offered to a broader spectrum of patients as surgeons become more comfortable with the procedure (**Figures 5** and **6**).

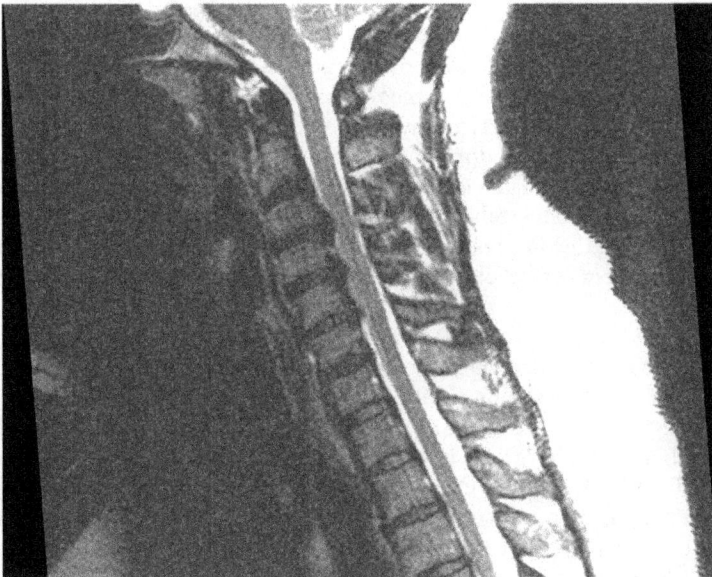

Figure 5.
Sagittal T2 MRI of a 38-year-old woman with worsening neck pain and radiculopathy. Note multi-level cervical disc herniations with cord impingement. Given her age, nerve impingement, isolated soft tissue pathology, and failure of conservative care patient was an ideal candidate for three-level cervical arthroplasty.

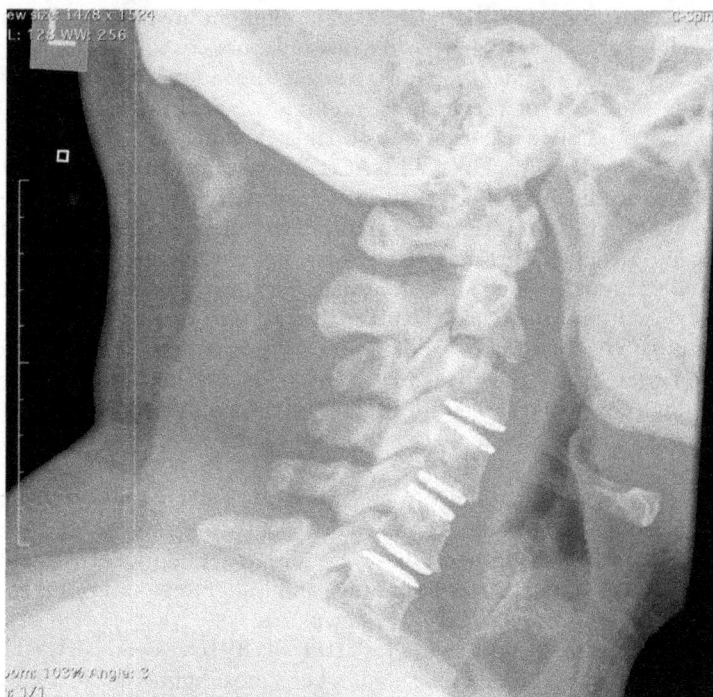

Figure 6.
Post-op lateral cervical spine x-ray demonstrating some restoration of lordosis and Orthofix M-6 arthroplasty devices at C3–4, C4–5, and C5–6.

9. Pearls

Early in the Globus Secure-C study [40], we observed some heterotopic ossification in spite of oral NSAIDs. This led many surgeons to try additional measures to reduce this phenomenon. Several surgeons sealed the anterior edges of the adjoining bodies with bone wax, particularly where the anterior longitudinal ligament was denuded from the bone. Anecdotally, this appeared to reduce the incidence of HO.

In my experience, I've had a lower rate of autofusion by incorporating the same technique along the uncovertebral joints. The proximity of neighboring bone in this area after aggressive decompression puts it at risk for heterotopic bone formation. As such I seal the areas of decorticated bone with a thin layer of bone wax even into the joint.

Many devices have keels or teeth that provide initial fixation. I often "set" the implant into the neighboring bone by compressing the implant using the Caspar pins in compression. This helps reduce overdistraction of the facets as well.

When using a keel-based implant such as ProDisc, I recommend using the mill rather than chiseling. There have been case reports [41, 42] of fractures of the vertebral body using the chisel even in the low-profile Prestige-LP [43]. Similar findings have occurred in lumbar cases with ProDisc-L. [44] where there is no milling rig available. Concern over fractures like these should be even greater in multilevel cases [45]. Interestingly, all of these cases used the bone chisels to make the keel cut. While there is no data to support the use of the milling bit, it appears to be a less invasive option (**Figure** 7).

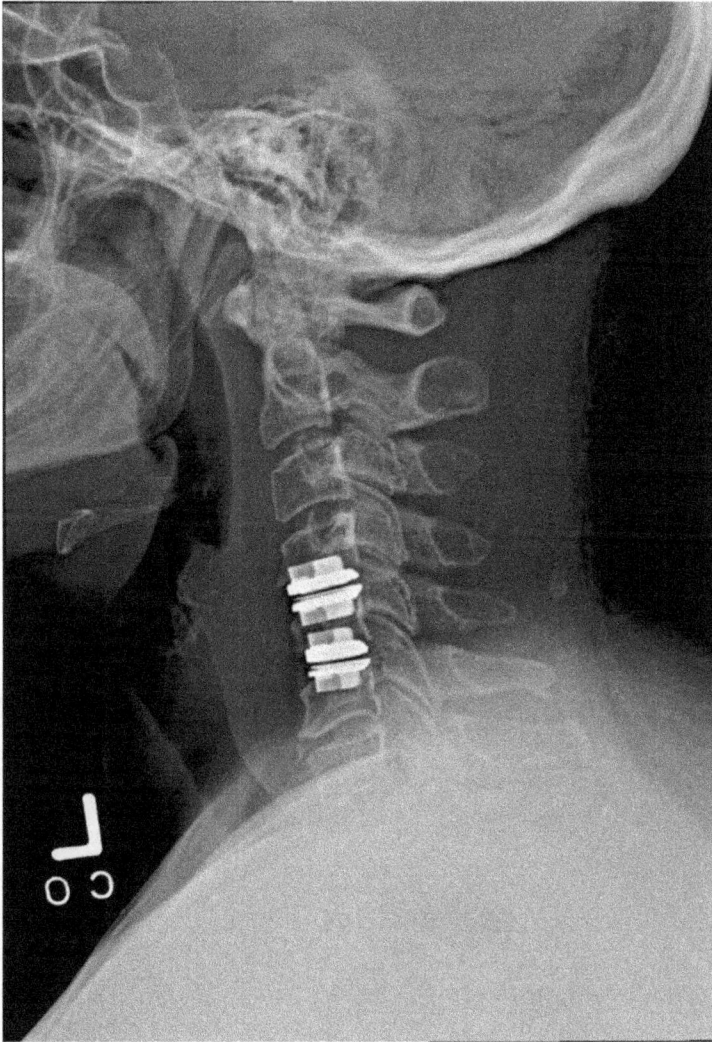

Figure 7.
Long keels on the Centinel spine ProDisc-C illustrate the intervening vertebral body compromise in patients with short vertebral bodies.

10. Future design implications

A number of other implant designs have been proposed albeit with little clinical implementation. The hydrogel Prosthetic Disc Nucleus (PDN) is a hydrogel core in a polyethylene shell or jacket meant to only replace the nucleus in the lumbar spine while preserving the annulus fibrosis. This technique relied on the compressed core to be inserted and absorb fluid over the first four or five days allowing it to expand and restore disc height. In the trend toward minimally invasive, there is great potential to become percutaneous. While stem cells have proven useful in osteobiologics, there is still a great need for their development in cartilage and disc replacement. Clearly, the future lies in cellular-based disc repair and reconstruction but for now, that hope is elusive.

Author details

Jason M. Highsmith
Carolina Neurosurgery and Orthopedics, Charleston, SC, USA

*Address all correspondence to: jhighsmith@yahoo.com

IntechOpen

References

[1] Probst C. Lumbar disk hernia: Microsurgery--yes or no? Neurochirurgia. 1989;**32**(6):172-176

[2] Henderson CM, Hennessy RG, Shuey HM Jr, Shackelford EG. Posterior-lateral foraminotomy as an exclusive operative technique for cervical radiculopathy: A review of 846 consecutively operated cases. Neurosurgery. 1983;**13**(5):504-512

[3] Adamson TE. Microendoscopic posterior cervical laminoforaminotomy for unilateral radiculopathy:Results of a new technique in 100 cases. Journal of Neurosurgery. 2001;**95**(Suppl. 1):51-57

[4] Jho H-D. Anterior microforaminotomy for cervical radiculopathy: A disc preservation technique. In: Neurosurgery Operative Color Atlas. Baltimore: Williams & Wilkins; 1998. pp. 43-52

[5] Jho HD, Kim WK, Kim MH. Anterior microforaminotomy for treatment of cervical radiculopathy: Part 1--disc-preserving "functional cervical disc surgery". Neurosurgery. 2002;**51**(Suppl. 5):S46-S53

[6] MacDowall A, Heary RF, Holy M, Lindhagen L, Olerud C. Posterior foraminotomy versus anterior decompression and fusion in patients with cervical degenerative disc disease with radiculopathy: Up to 5 years of outcome from the national Swedish spine register. Journal of Neurosurgery. Spine. 2019;**32**(3):1-9

[7] Robinson RA, Smith GW. Antero-lateral cervical disc removal and interbody fusion for cervical disc syndrome. (abstract.). Bulletin of the Johns Hopkins Hospital. 1955;**96**:223-224

[8] Cloward RB. The anterior approach for removal of ruptured cervical disks. Journal of Neurosurgery. 1958;**15**(6):602-617

[9] Heidecke V, Rainov NG, Marx T, Burkert W. Outcome in Cloward anterior fusion for degenerative cervical spinal disease. Acta Neurochirurgica. 2000;**142**(3):283-291

[10] Martin R, Carda JR, Pinto JI, Sanz F, Montiaga F, Paternina B, et al. Anterior cervical diskectomy and interbody arthrodesis using Cloward technique: Retrospective study of complications and radiological results of 167 cases. Neurocirugía (Asturias, Spain). 2002;**13**(4):265-284

[11] Vavruch L, Hedlund R, Javid D, Leszniewski W, Shalabi A. A prospective randomized comparison between the cloward procedure and a carbon fiber cage in the cervical spine: A clinical and radiologic study. Spine. 2002;**27**(16):1694-1701

[12] Smith GW, Robinson RA. The treatment of certain cervical-spine disorders by anterior removal of the intervertebral disc and interbody fusion. The Journal of Bone and Joint Surgery. American Volume 1958;40-A(3):607-624.

[13] Peolsson A, Peolsson M. Predictive factors for long-term outcome of anterior cervical decompression and fusion: A multivariate data analysis. European Spine Journal. 2008;**17**(3):406-414

[14] Rehman L, Qayoom Khan HA, Hashim AS. Outcome of Cloward technique in cervical disc prolapse. Journal of the College of Physicians and Surgeons–Pakistan. 2010;**20**(11):733-737

[15] Noriega DC, Kreuger A, Brotat M, Ardura F, Hernandez R, Munoz MF, et al. Long-term outcome of the Cloward procedure for single-level cervical degenerative spondylosis. Clinical and radiological assessment after a 22-year mean follow-up.

Acta Neurochirurgica. 2013;**155**(12): 2339-2344

[16] Fernyhough JC, Schimandle JJ, Weigel MC, Edwards CC, Levine AM. Chronic donor site pain complicating bone graft harvesting from the posterior iliac crest for spinal fusion. Spine. 1992;**17**(12):1474-1480

[17] Dial BL, Esposito VR, Danilkowicz R, O'Donnell J, Sugarman B, Blizzard DJ, et al. Factors associated with extended length of stay and 90-day readmission rates following ACDF. Global Spine Journal. 2020;**10**(3):252-260

[18] Lind BI, Zoega B, Rosen H. Autograft versus interbody fusion cage without plate fixation in the cervical spine: A randomized clinical study using radiostereometry. European Spine Journal. 2007;**16**(8):1251-1256

[19] Jain A, Marrache M, Harris A, Puvanesarajah V, Neuman BJ, Buser Z, et al. Structural allograft versus PEEK implants in anterior cervical discectomy and fusion: A systematic review. Global Spine Journal. 2020;**10**(6):775-783

[20] Fransen P. A simplified technique for anterior cervical discectomy and fusion using a screw-plate implanted over the Caspar distractor pins. Acta Orthopaedica Belgica. 2010;**76**(4): 546-548

[21] Dumont TM, Lin CT, Tranmer BI, Horgan MA. Pseudarthrosis failures of anterior subaxial cervical spine fusion using a plate with a single screw per vertebral body: A case series. World Neurosurgery. 2014;**82**(1-2):225-230

[22] Gabr MA, Touko E, Yadav AP, Karikari I, Goodwin CR, Groff MW, et al. Improved dysphagia outcomes in anchored spacers versus plate-screw systems in anterior cervical discectomy and fusion: A systematic review. Global Spine Journal. 2020;**10**(8):1057-1065

[23] Findlay LC, Beasley E, Park J, Kohen DE, Algan Y, Vitaro F, et al. Longitudinal child data: What can be gained by linking administrative data and cohort data? International Journal of Population Data Science. 2018;**3**(1):451

[24] Lee YS, Kim YB, Park SW. Does a zero-profile anchored cage offer additional stabilization as anterior cervical plate? Spine. 2015;**40**(10): E563-E570

[25] Hofstetter CP, Kesavabhotla K, Boockvar JA. Zero-profile anchored spacer reduces rate of dysphagia compared with ACDF with anterior plating. Journal of Spinal Disorders & Techniques. 2015;**28**(5):E284-E290

[26] Basu S, Rathinavelu S. A prospective study of clinical and radiological outcomes of zero-profile cage screw implants for single-level anterior cervical discectomy and fusion: Is segmental lordosis maintained at 2 years? Asian Spine Journal. 2017;**11**(2):264-271

[27] Kang DG, Wagner SC, Tracey RW, Cody JP, Gaume RE, Lehman RA Jr. Biomechanical stability of a stand-alone interbody spacer in two-level and hybrid cervical fusion constructs. Global Spine Journal. 2017;7(7):681-688

[28] Chang UK, Kim DH, Lee MC, Willenberg R, Kim SH, Lim J. Changes in adjacent-level disc pressure and facet joint force after cervical arthroplasty compared with cervical discectomy and fusion. Journal of Neurosurgery. Spine. 2007;7(1):33-39

[29] Chen J, Fan SW, Wang XW, Yuan W. Motion analysis of single-level cervical total disc arthroplasty: A meta-analysis. Orthopaedic Surgery. 2012;**4**(2):94-100

[30] Dmitriev AE, Cunningham BW, Hu N, Sell G, Vigna F, McAfee PC. Adjacent level intradiscal pressure and

segmental kinematics following a cervical total disc arthroplasty: An in vitro human cadaveric model. Spine. 2005;**30**(10):1165-1172

[31] Robertson JT, Papadopoulos SM, Traynelis VC. Assessment of adjacent-segment disease in patients treated with cervical fusion or arthroplasty: A prospective 2-year study. Journal of Neurosurgery. Spine. 2005;**3**(6):417-423

[32] Lopez-Espina CG, Amirouche F, Havalad V. Multilevel cervical fusion and its effect on disc degeneration and osteophyte formation. Spine. 2006;**31**(9):972-978

[33] Swank ML, Lowery GL, Bhat AL, McDonough RF. Anterior cervical allograft arthrodesis and instrumentation: Multilevel interbody grafting or strut graft reconstruction. European Spine Journal. 1997;**6**(2):138-143

[34] Veeravagu A, Cole T, Jiang B, Ratliff JK. Revision rates and complication incidence in single- and multilevel anterior cervical discectomy and fusion procedures: An administrative database study. The Spine Journal. 2014;**14**(7):1125-1131

[35] Fernstrom U. Arthroplasty with intercorporal endoprothesis in herniated disc and in painful disc. Acta Chirurgica Scandinavica. Supplementum. 1966;**357**:154-159

[36] Alemo-Hammad S. Use of acrylic in anterior cervical discectomy: Technical note. Neurosurgery. 1985;**17**(1):94-96

[37] Cummins BH, Robertson JT, Gill SS. Surgical experience with an implanted artificial cervical joint. Journal of Neurosurgery. 1998;**88**(6):943-948

[38] Kerferd JW, Abi-Hanna D, Phan K, Rao P, Mobbs RJ. Focal hypermobility observed in cervical arthroplasty with Mobi-C. Journal of Spine Surgery. 2017;**3**(4):693-696

[39] DiCesare JAT, Tucker AM, Say I, Patel K, Lanman TH, Coufal FJ, et al. Mechanical failure of the Mobi-C implant for artificial cervical disc replacement: Report of 4 cases. Journal of Neurosurgery. Spine. 2020;**33**(6):751-756

[40] Vaccaro A, Beutler W, Peppelman W, Marzluff JM, Highsmith J, Mugglin A, et al. Clinical outcomes with selectively constrained SECURE-C cervical disc arthroplasty: Two-year results from a prospective, randomized, controlled, multicenter investigational device exemption study. Spine. 2013;**38**(26):2227-2239

[41] Shim CS, Shin HD, Lee SH. Posterior avulsion fracture at adjacent vertebral body during cervical disc replacement with ProDisc-C: A case report. Journal of Spinal Disorders & Techniques. 2007;**20**(6):468-472

[42] Anderson PA, Sasso RC, Hipp J, Norvell DC, Raich A, Hashimoto R. Kinematics of the cervical adjacent segments after disc arthroplasty compared with anterior discectomy and fusion: A systematic review and meta-analysis. Spine. 2012;**37**(Suppl. 22): S85-S95

[43] Dong L, Wang D, Chen X, Liu T, Xu Z, Tan M, et al. A comprehensive meta-analysis of the adjacent segment parameters in cervical disk arthroplasty versus anterior cervical discectomy and fusion. Clinical Spine Surgery. 2018;**31**(4):162-173

[44] Shim CS, Lee S, Maeng DH, Lee SH. Vertical split fracture of the vertebral body following total disc replacement using ProDisc: Report of two cases. Journal of Spinal Disorders & Techniques. 2005;**18**(5):465-469

[45] Datta JC, Janssen ME, Beckham R, Ponce C. Sagittal split fractures in multilevel cervical arthroplasty using a keeled prosthesis. Journal of Spinal Disorders & Techniques. 2007;**20**(1): 89-92

Chapter 4

Safety and Efficiency of Cervical Disc Arthroplasty in Ambulatory Surgery Centers

Richard N.W. Wohns

Abstract

Introduction Anterior cervical surgeries have been safely performed in ambulatory surgery centers since 1995 with the first cases being one level anterior cervical discectomies without fusion, then in 1996, one level anterior cervical discectomies with fusion (ACDF). When it is was certain that outpatient fusion was safe, the number of ACDF levels slowly and methodically were increased to the now standard outpatient maximum of four level ACDF. During this evolution, with the introduction of arthroplasty surgery, one level arthroplasties were considered appropriate for outpatient surgery and now two-level outpatient cervical arthroplasties are routine and some three level arthroplasties have been performed with no additional morbidity compared to one level procedures. The author first reported a series of 27 patients in 2010 who underwent cervical disc replacement at an ASC. (Wohns, R. Safety and cost-effectiveness of outpatient cervical disc arthroplasty. Surg. Neurol. Int. 1, 77, 2010). The average operative time was 40 minutes and the patients were observed over a period of three hours prior to discharge. None of the patients had major complications and there were no reports of worsening or persistent pain. The results of a Delphi study in 2018 compared the safety and efficiency of one-level and two-level arthroplasty procedures performed in an ASC and in a hospital setting. (Gornet et al. Safety and Efficiency of Cervical Disc Arthroplasty in Ambulatory Surgery Centers vs Hospital Settings. Int'l J of Spine Surgery. Vol. 12, No.5, 2018, pp. 557-564). The study analyzed outcomes of 145 ASC patients, 348 hospital outpatients and 65 hospital inpatients and the conclusion was that both one and two-level arthroplasties may be performed safely in an ASC. Surgeries in ASCs are of shorter duration and performed with less blood loss without increased AEs. At the present time, there does not appear to be any contraindication to performing the vast majority of cervical arthroplasties in an ambulatory surgery center (ASC). Furthermore, the cost of an outpatient arthroplasty is commonly 30% to 50% of the cost of hospital-based procedures.

Keywords: Outpatient, cervical disc arthroplasty, ASC, ambulatory surgery center

1. Introduction

Anterior cervical surgeries have been safely performed in ambulatory surgery centers since 1995 with the first cases being one level anterior cervical discectomies without fusion, then in 1996, one level anterior cervical discectomies with fusion

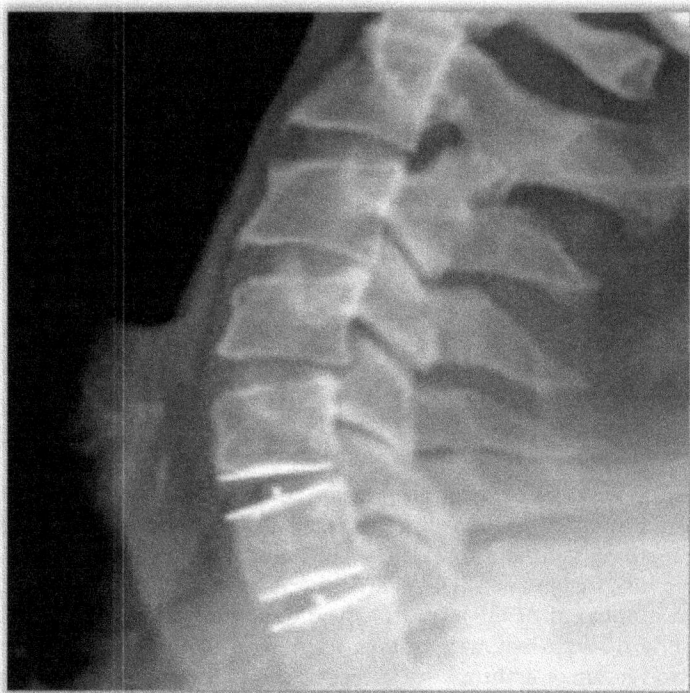

Figure 1.
Lateral cervical x-ray showing successful two-level arthroplasty (C5-6, C6-7).

(ACDF) [1]. When it is was certain that outpatient fusion was safe, the number of ACDF levels slowly and methodically were increased to the now standard outpatient maximum of four level ACDF. During this evolution, with the introduction of arthroplasty surgery, one level arthroplasties were considered appropriate for outpatient surgery and now two-level outpatient cervical arthroplasties are routine and some three level arthroplasties have been performed with no additional morbidity compared to one level procedures. The author first reported a series of 27 patients in 2010 who underwent cervical disc replacement at an ASC [2]. The average operative time was 40 minutes and the patients were observed over a period of three hours prior to discharge. None of the patients had major complications and there were no reports of worsening or persistent pain. The results of a Delphi study in 2018 compared the safety and efficiency of one-level and two-level arthroplasty procedures performed in an ASC and in a hospital setting [3]. The study analyzed outcomes of 145 ASC patients, 348 hospital outpatients and 65 hospital inpatients and the conclusion was that both one and two-level arthroplasties may be performed safely in an ASC. Surgeries in ASCs are of shorter duration and performed with less blood loss without increased AEs. At the present time, there does not appear to be any contra-indication to performing the vast majority of cervical arthroplasties in an ambulatory surgery center (ASC). Furthermore, the cost of an outpatient arthroplasty is commonly 30–50% of the cost of hospital-based procedures (**Figure 1**).

Indications for Cervical Arthroplasty.

The indications for arthroplasty vs. fusion are the same regardless of site of service, i.e., hospital inpatient, hospital outpatient (HOPD) vs. ASC outpatient. These indications include the following:

1. Skeletally mature patients

2. One or two contiguous levels (C3-7) for intractable radiculopathy with or without neck pain or myelopathy due to abnormality localized to the level of the disc space

3. Axial cervical pain due to discogenic etiology, proven with concordant discography

4. At least one of the following confirmed by MRI or CT/myelogram:

   a. Herniated nucleus pulposus

   b. Spondylosis with or without Modic endplate changes

   c. Visible loss of disc height compared to adjacent levels

5. Failure of at least six weeks of conservative treatment or progressive signs or symptoms despite non-operative treatment

2. Contraindications for cervical arthroplasty

The contraindications for arthroplasty vs. fusion are the same regardless of site of service, i.e., hospital inpatient, hospital outpatient (HOPD) vs. ASC outpatient, with the exception of certain medical co-morbidities which would preclude safe outpatient surgery. The medical co-morbidities that would require hospital inpatient arthroplasty include the following:

1. Anti-coagulation that cannot be safely discontinued peri-operatively, and therefore bridge anti-coagulation is required

2. Brittle diabetes

3. Significant sleep apnea requiring CPAP

4. Lack of proper post-operative home support by family or friends

5. Chronic opioid dependence with daily morphine equivalent >60

Otherwise, the routine contraindications for arthroplasty, regardless of site of service are the following:

1. Acute or chronic infection, systemic or at the operative site

2. Known allergy or sensitivity to the implant materials (cobalt, chromium, molybdenum, titanium, hydroxyapatite, or polyethylene)

3. Compromised vertebral bodies at the index level (e.g., ankylosing spondylitis, rheumatoid arthritis)

4. Marked cervical instability on resting lateral or flexion-extension x-rays

5. Osteoporosis or osteopenia (DEXA DMB T-score < −1.5)

6. Severe facet joint disease or degeneration

3. Post-operative care following cervical arthroplasty

The post-operative care following arthroplasty is the same regardless of site of service, i.e., hospital inpatient, hospital outpatient (HOPD) vs. ASC outpatient, with the exception of the length of stay i.e. time to discharge post-operatively. In the ASC setting, the time to discharge is three hours whereas the time to discharge in a hospital setting may be 24-48 hours. The care includes the following:

1. Ambulate the day of surgery

2. No lifting, bending (particularly extension), twisting x 4 weeks

3. Soft collar for use only in a car x 4 weeks

4. Meloxicam x 3 weeks

5. Back to work 1-2 weeks

6. Physical therapy, including:

    a. Isometric strengthening typically at 2 weeks

    b. Dynamic range of motion at 6 weeks as needed

7. Restrict overhead activity, repetitive neck movements, and heavy lifting for 6 weeks

4. Clinical benefits of arthroplasty vs. fusion

Cervical arthroplasty is designed to provide maintenance of physiologic motion and prevent or mitigate the negative sequelae of fusion as follows:

1. Up to 3.5 times less radiographic adjacent level degeneration

2. Nearly 4 times fewer re-operations

3. Up to 16.5% better disability improvement

4. Maintenance of motion up to 10 years post-operative

5. Up to 3 weeks faster return to work

5. Surgical technique

When cervical arthroplasty devices were first FDA approved and released on the market, it was presumed by this author that the procedure would be as safe or safer

Surgery Levels	2013	2014	2015	2016	2017	2018	2019	2020
1	14	30	34	38	37	40	47	11
2			6	3	12	27	37	12
Total	14	30	40	41	49	67	84	23

Figure 2.
Table graph showing the author's number of outpatient cervical arthroplasties from 2013 through 2020.

than ACDF for several reasons. The majority of patients who undergo arthroplasty rather than fusion do not require use of a drill with resulting bone bleeding. The arthroplasty procedure is performed with removal of the cartilaginous endplates but not the bony endplates. The result is less bleeding and an overall faster procedure than ACDF surgery. Otherwise, the arthroplasty procedure is very similar to an ACDF. There have been numerous papers proving safety and efficiency of outpatient ACDF surgery [4, 5].

In the author's personal experience of more than 400 outpatient arthroplasties including both one- and two-level procedures, there have been no major AEs (**Figure 2**).

Author details

Richard N.W. Wohns[1,2,3]

1 NeoSpine, Washington, USA

2 University of Washington, Seattle, Washington, USA

3 Tribhuvan University Teaching Hospital, Kathmandu, Nepal

*Address all correspondence to: rwohns@wohnsconsultinggroup.com

IntechOpen

References

[1] Wohns, RNW (1999): Outpatient Anterior Cervical Microdiscectomy: Experience with 106 cases. Ambulatory Surgery 7:35-37

[2] Wohns, R (2010). Safety and cost-effectiveness of outpatient cervical disc arthroplasty. Surg. Neurol. Int. **1,** 77, 2010

[3] Gornet (2018). Safety and Efficiency of Cervical Disc Arthroplasty in Ambulatory Surgery Centers vs Hospital Settings. Int'l J of Spine Surgery. **Vol. 12,** No.5, pp. 557-564

[4] Joseffer (2010) Outpatient anterior cervical discectomy and fusion: indications and clinical experience in a consecutive series of 390 patients. Neurosurg Quarterly; 20(2): 10-110

[5] Villavicencio (2007). The safety of instrumented outpatient anterior cervical discectomy and fusion. Spine J; 7(2):148-153

Section 2

Minimally Invasive
Thoracic Approaches

Chapter 5

Minimally Invasive Lateral Approach for Anterior Spinal Cord Decompression in Thoracic Myelopathy

Edna E. Gouveia, Mansour Mathkour, Erin McCormack,
Jonathan Riffle, Olawale A. Sulaiman and Daniel J. Denis

Abstract

Myelopathy can result from a thoracic disc herniation (TDH) compressing the anterior spinal cord. Disc calcification and difficulty in accessing the anterior spinal cord pose an operative challenge. A mini-open lateral approach to directly decompress the anterior spinal cord can be performed with or without concomitant interbody fusion depending on pre-existing or iatrogenic spinal instability. Experience using stand-alone expandable spacers to achieve interbody fusion in this setting is limited. Technical advantages, risks and limitations of this technique are discussed. We conducted a retrospective chart review of all patients with thoracic and upper lumbar myelopathy treated with a lateral mini-open lateral approach. Review of the literature identified 6 other case series using similar lateral minimally invasive approaches to treat thoracic or upper lumbar disc herniation showing efficient and safe thoracic disc decompression procedure for myelopathy. This technique can be combined with interbody arthrodesis when instability is suspected.

Keywords: Expandable, interbody, lateral, minimally invasive, thoracic myelopathy

1. Introduction

Rapidly progressing myelopathy can result from a thoracic or upper lumbar disc herniation compressing the anterior spinal cord. With a prevalence of approximately 6.5%, thoracic disc herniation (TDH) is not routinely diagnosed [1]. This low incidence contributes to the lack of familiarity with treatment methods and several factors contribute to a reticence for treating TDH. The calcified or ossified nature of the pathology, the difficulty to safely access and decompress the anterior spinal cord without causing worsening myelopathy and the complications associated with thoracic or thoracolumbar spinal approaches make this condition challenging for the spine surgeon.

The anterior thoracotomy approach has been traditionally considered as a treatment of choice to treat thoracic disc pathology. Compared to the posterior approaches, such as the costotransversectomy, anterior approaches can offer increased visualization and access to safely decompress midline thoracic lesions. To minimize pain and pulmonary complications associated with thoracotomy, thoracoscopic [2] and more recently the lateral mini-open technique have been reported to treat thoracic disc pathology [3–9]. Although considered a lateral approach, this technique offer direct access to the anterior spinal canal without requiring retraction of the dural sac. Another significant advantage of the lateral mini-open approach is it can be performed without depending on a thoracic access surgeon.

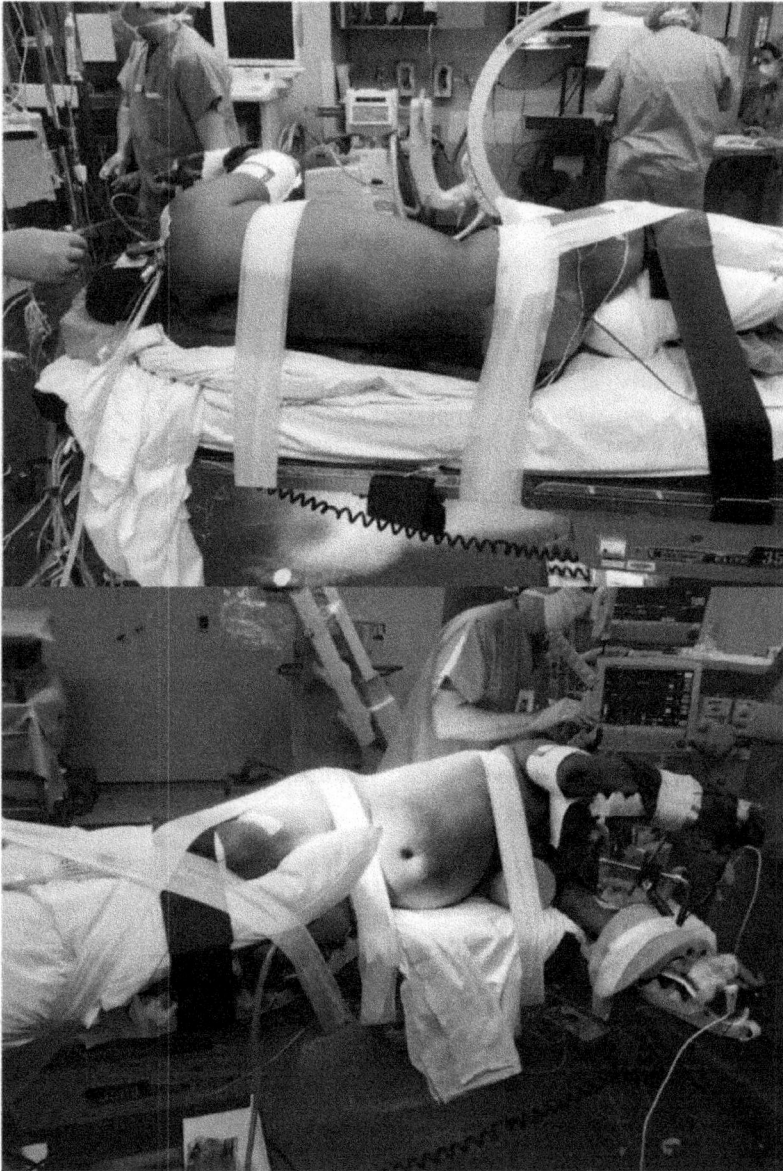

Figure 1.
The lateral decubitus position was used for the thoracic mini-open lateral approach in a patient with T10–11 myelopathy. Note that the tape used to secure the upper body should be positioned closer to the shoulders in the case of a more rostral thoracic spinal level.

2. Surgical procedure

Under general anesthesia and without dual-lumen intubation, patients are positioned on lateral decubitus (**Figure 1**). Motor and sensory evoked potentials are monitored intraoperatively. A left or right side approach is chosen to access the same side of the disc protrusion if lateralized. Careful preoperative review of thoracic spine computed tomography (CT) and/or magnetic resonance imaging (MRI) helped localize the large vessels. Pre-operative hook-wire localization can be performed to accurately localize the pathology [4]. For midline anterior lesions, the senior author prefers a right-sided approach to avoid the descending aorta from T5–6 to T8–9. The location of the descending aorta on the left side of the vertebral body from T5 to T8 needs to be taken into account if the contralateral annulus needs to be released during the interbody arthrodesis. Breaking the table is usually not performed.

Under fluoroscopic localization, the anterior and posterior limit of the vertebral bodies above and below the pathological level are delineated. A 3–5 cm incision must span the entire anteroposterior distance of the disc space and is extended posteriorly over or between the underlying ribs. After blunt dissection of the intercostal muscles the rib is partially resected using Leksell and/or Kerrisons rongeurs. The bone is kept as autograft or can be replaced using rib reconstruction techniques to reduce intercostal wound pain. The retropleural space is then dissected bluntly by retracting the parietal pleura from the thoracic wall using sponge sticks or endoscopic kittners. Further rib resection posteriorly may help the dissection if needed. The rib head is then palpated in the retropleural space. Serial dilators are inserted and the retractor blade length is chosen. Using fluoroscopy in lateral

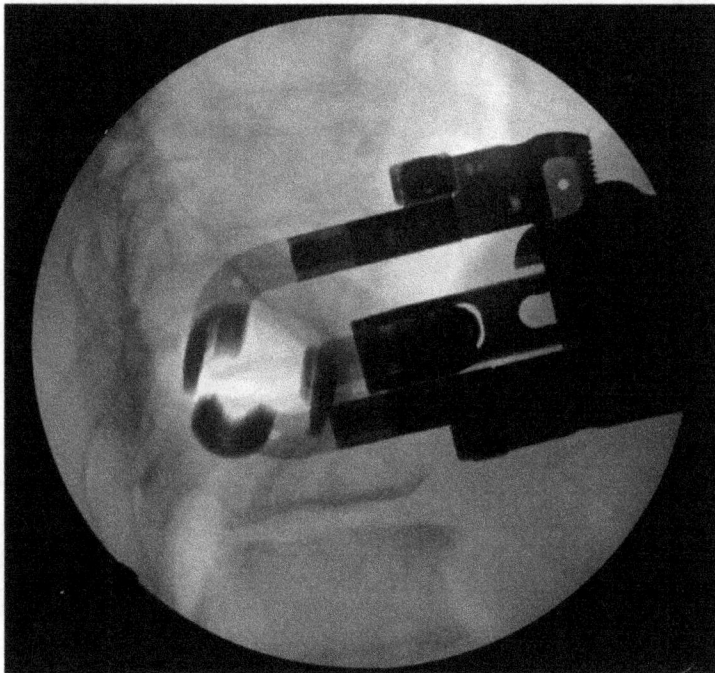

Figure 2.
Intraoperative fluoroscopic image showing positioning of the retractor. The working space is centered over the posterior disc space and the anterior spinal canal junction.

projection the table-mounted 3 blade retractors are centered at the junction of the posterior disc and the canal (**Figure 2**). The middle blade is oriented anteriorly toward the lung to retract the parietal pleura. This leaves a space between the caudal and cranial blades where instruments can be freely manipulated (**Figure 3**). In the case where the parietal pleural is inadvertently torn and the lung is visualized, the approach becomes transthoracic and a placement of a laparotomy compress between the lung and the middle blade aids with exposure as well as protects the visceral pleura.

Using the operating microscope or loupes with a headlight, the parietal pleura over the rib head and disc space is divided using a long tip cautery tool. Careful attention is aimed at preserving the exiting nerve root. When identified, the exiting nerve root can be retracted and protected with the cranial blade of the retractor. Using a high-speed drill with 16-cm minimally invasive curve attachments (Stryker, Kalamazoo, MI), the rib head is drilled and bony struts are created in the

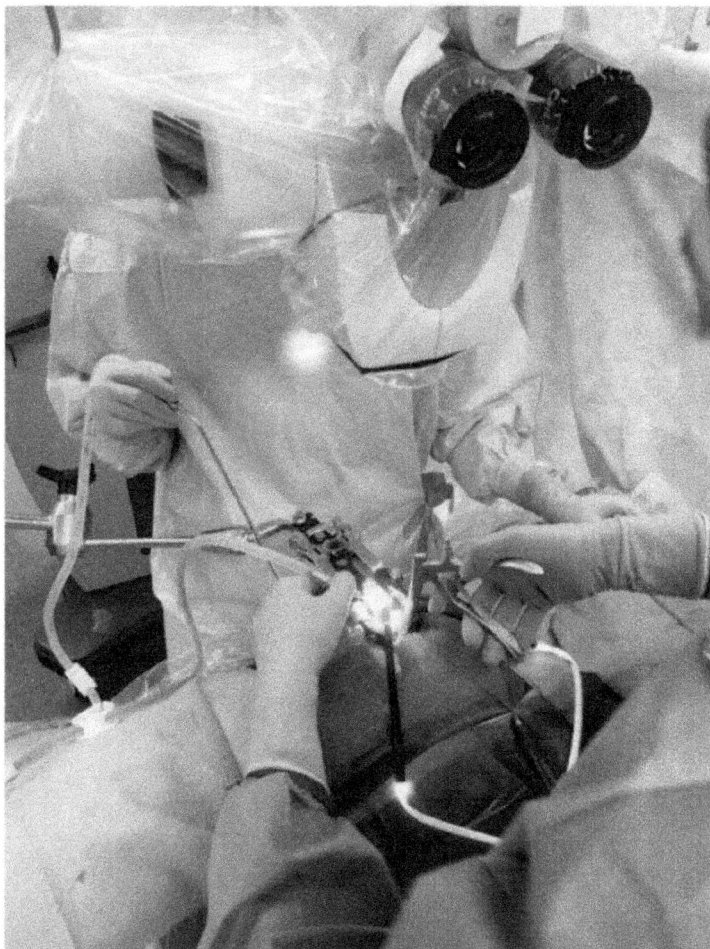

Figure 3.
Left-sided approach. The surgeon is facing the back of the patient. The patient head is to the right side of the picture. The orthostatic retractor is positioned with the middle blade retracting the parietal pleural and lung away from the surgeon. Instruments are manipulated between the caudal and rostral blades.

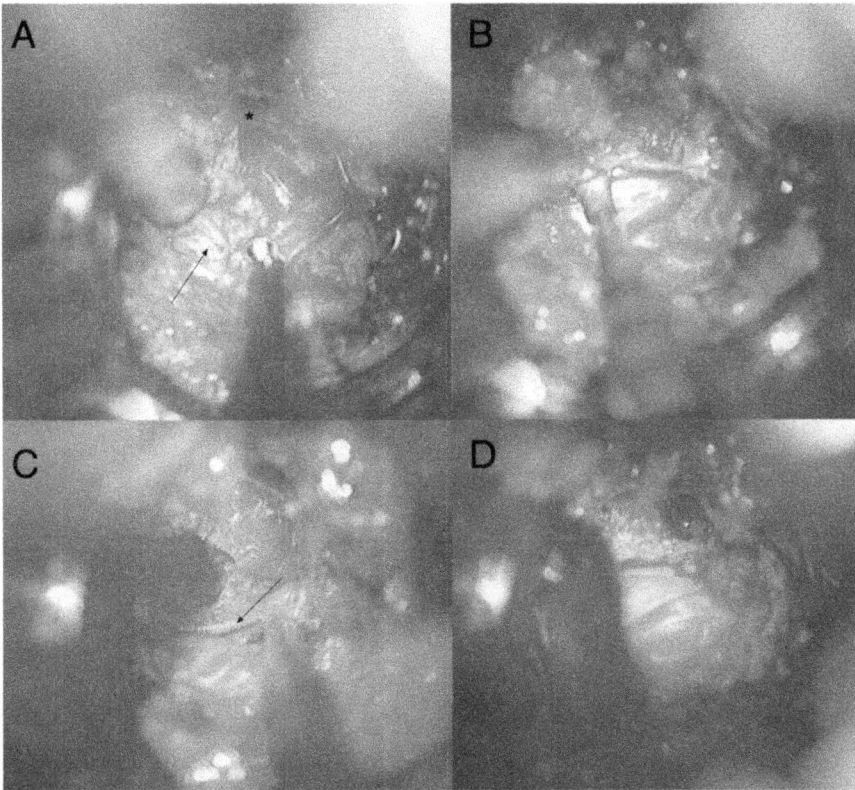

Figure 4.
Intraoperative images under microscopic visualization. A: The rib head has been resected and bony struts (*) have been drilled to delineate the posterior disc space. A soft disc herniation (arrow) is encountered once the spinal canal is entered. B: The dura become more apparent and discectomy anterior to the dura is carried out. C: A curved curette is placed between the posterior longitudinal ligament (arrow) and the anterior dural sac. D: The anterior dura has been decompressed.

vertebral bodies on each side of the posterior disc space to create a partial corpectomy space where disc fragments can be dislodged without retracting the dural sac. Drilling of the superior pedicle of the inferior vertebral body helps to expose the spinal canal. The posterior disc is removed with pituitary rongeurs. Ossified disc herniations are drilled laterally just anterior to the dural sac until they become completely freed from the vertebral bodies and disc space. Then the remaining osteophytes can be gently dissected from the posterior longitudinal ligament (PLL) and dura in the partial corpectomy space without excessive manipulation of the spinal cord (**Figure 4**). Resection of the PLL helps to visualize the dura to assess the decompression. Once the dural sac is fully decompressed anteriorly, an interbody arthrodesis can be accomplished by mobilizing the retractor in the center of the disc space in the anteroposterior plane. The discectomy can then be completed with serial shavers. The contralateral annulus can be released with a Cobb elevator in order to place an interbody cage which spans the full apophyseal ring of the vertebral bodies. An expandable stand-alone cage (Rise-L, Globus Medical, Audubon, PA, USA) filled with autograft and allograft is then positioned. A Jackson-Pratt or Hemovac drain is left in the retropleural or intrapleural cavity. In the event of a visceral pleura laceration, placement of a chest tube is preferred (**Figures 5–7**).

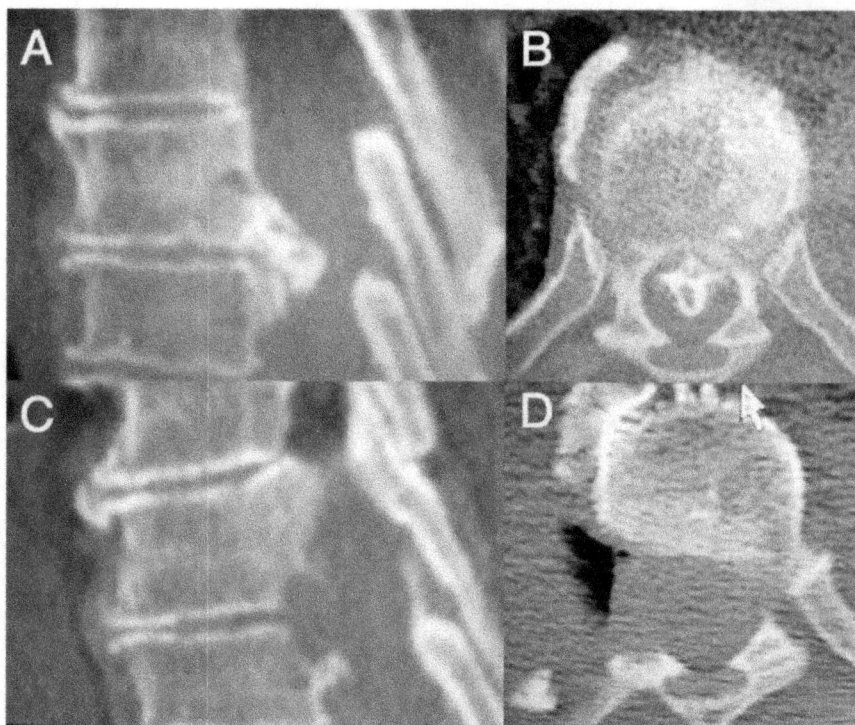

Figure 5.
Preoperative sagittal (A) and axial (B) computed tomography images show an ossified disc herniation at T7–8 in a 72 years old female. Post-operative images (C-D) show complete decompression of the spinal canal.

3. Experience and review of literature

This technique has been preferred by the author to treat one or two levels thoracic myelopathy. A total of 15 consecutive cases, 73% males and 27% females, who underwent a thoracic or thoracolumbar lateral mini-open approach to decompress the anterior spinal canal were included (**Table 1**). Mean age at surgery was 55.8 years (range, 38–76) and mean body mass index was 33.8 kg/m^2 (range, 22.8–50.9). Fourteen patients presented with myelopathy symptoms while only six patients presented with radicular thoracic pain. A calcified disc was found in two patients. The most frequent level affected was T10–11. Two patients had two consecutive levels treated. Mean estimated blood loss was 400 mL (range, 50–2150) and mean operative time was 188 minutes (range, 113–328). Mean length of stay was 8 days (range, 2–23). No positive correlation was found between BMI and ORT, $r = 0.2392$, $p = 0.2073$. Elective surgery was performed in 8 cases with a mean length of stay of 4 days (range, 2–9). At a mean follow-up of 11.1 months, myelopathy significantly improved in a majority of patients (**Tables 1** and **2**).

The mini-open direct lateral approach has gained popularity to perform indirect decompression and interbody fusion in the lumbar spine [10] (**Tables 3** and **4**). Below the L2–3 level, the direct lateral approach is usually not performed to directly decompress the spinal canal because placement of the retractor more dorsally can result in direct nerve injury due to the proximity of the lumbar plexus [9]. Above L1–2, the mini-open lateral approach can be safely performed to remove midline anterior lesions and directly decompress the spinal cord and ipsilateral exiting nerve

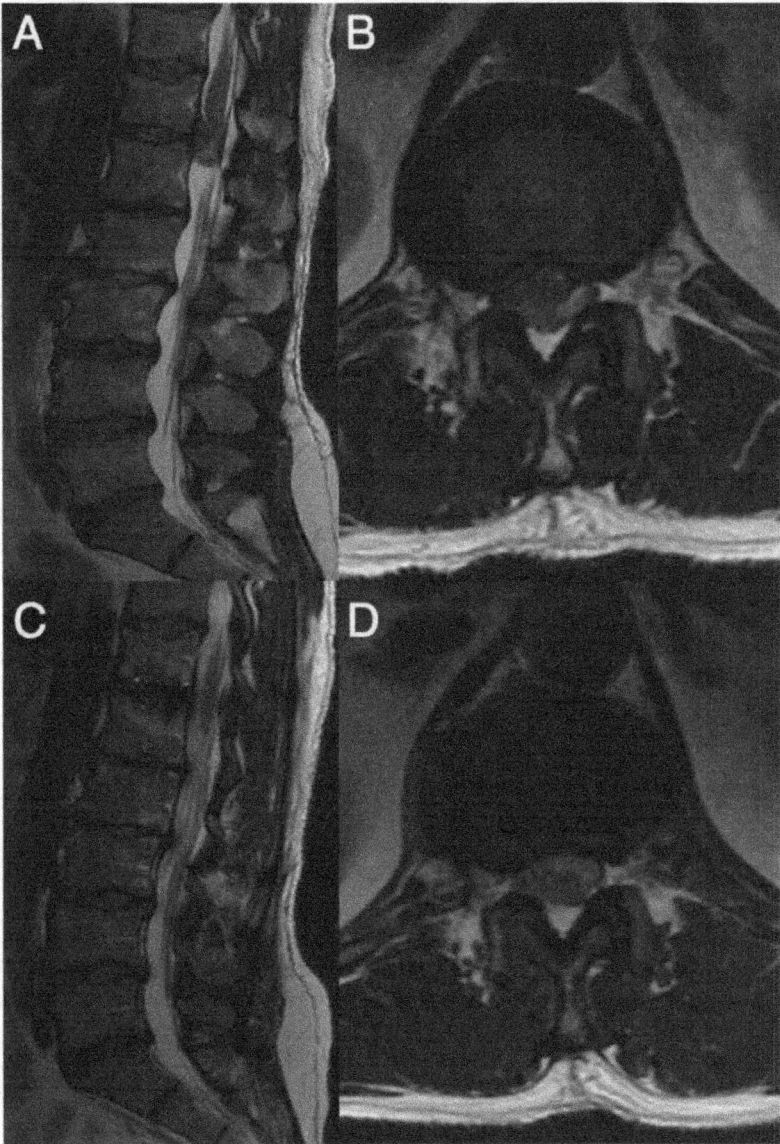

Figure 6.
Preoperative sagittal (A) and axial (B) T2-weighted magnetic resonance images of a soft disc herniation at T12-L1 in a 51 years old male. Post-operative images (C-D) show decompression of the spinal canal. Note that expandable cage artifacts do not affect interpretation.

root (**Table 5**). At L1–2 and L2–3, the author experience has shown this approach to be useful in decompressing the anterior spinal canal but special care needs to be taken to identify and protect the exiting nerve root.

3.1 Obesity and surgical outcomes

Obesity is a risk factor for lumbar spondylosis [11, 12] and prior studies suggest that class I obesity is frequently found in patients with symptomatic thoracic or thoracolumbar spondylosis [7, 9]. The mini-open lateral approach was found to be

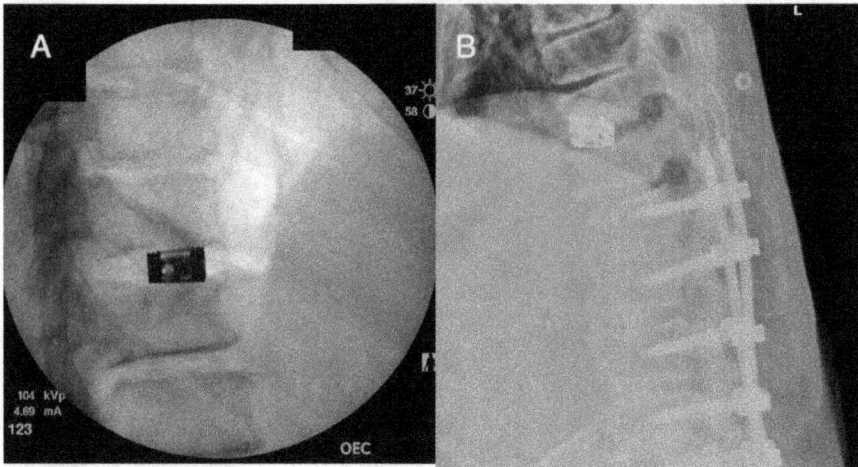

Figure 7.
A: Intra-operative fluoroscopy showing ideal placement of expandable interbody spacer (case no. 7). **B:**
Example of cage subsidence 6 weeks after surgery in case no. 13.

ideal in treating morbid obese patients as the amount of adipose tissue did not interfere with the approach (**Figure 8**). The working length is increased in obese patients, mandating usage of longer retractor blades, but the body mass index is not associated with increased surgical time.

3.2 Concomitant interbody arthrodesis and supplemental instrumentation

Delayed deformity following thoracic discectomy without instrumented fusion has been reported as low as <3% [13]. In the case of rapidly worsening myelopathy caused by extrusion of a soft or partially calcified thoracic disc, concomitant arthrodesis is often performed as the condition is thought to result from chronic instability [13, 14]. The extent of the decompression by removing the posterior longitudinal ligament (PLL), the ipsilateral inferior pedicle and/or the lateral facet complex can also potentially increase segmental instability. However the natural history and pathophysiology of TDH presenting with myelopathy is still poorly understood and large thoracoscopic series has been performed without arthrodesis with successful long-term outcomes [15, 16].

Expandable lateral interbody cages have been shown to provide immediate stability, limiting flexion, extension, lateral bending and axial rotation comparable to static cages [17]. The main advantage is considered to be the small cage height (7 mm) at implantation, which is thought to minimize vertebral endplate disruption thus potentially decreasing later implant subsidence. The use of BMP-2 for interbody arthrodesis or adding supplemental anterior or posterior instrumentation should be considered when pre-existing factors that can lead to pseudoarthosis are present.

The author prefers using expendable spacer to decrease the risk of device migration during insertion. Because the PLL is frequently divided during the decompression procedure, a larger static cage could accidentally slip posteriorly during placement in the kyphotic thoracic spine, resulting in cord compression. This risk is similar to anterior cage migration during implantation of static cages when anterior longitudinal ligament release is performed for deformity correction in the lumbar spine [18].

Case no.	Age	Sex	Smoker	BMI	Myel.	Rad.	Cal.	Level (s)	Trans.	Arthro.	EBL (ml)	ORT (min)	LOS (days)
1	72	Female	No	31.7	Yes	No	Yes	T7–8	No	No	2150	233	3
2	51	Male	No	29.0	Yes	Yes	No	T12–L1	No	Yes	200	263	4
3	43	Male	No	50.9	Yes	No	No	T10–11	No	Yes	750	328	11
4	53	Male	No	40.0	Yes	No	No	T11–12	No	Yes	350	134	12
5	71	Male	No	29.0	Yes	No	No	T10–11	Yes	Yes	100	182	9
6	39	Male	Yes	24.0	Yes	Yes	No	T9–10	Yes	Yes	250	163	2
7	57	Male	No	31.1	Yes	No	No	T11–12	No	Yes	75	195	2
8	50	Female	No	35.8	Yes	No	Yes	T9–10	No	Yes	50	156	3
9	41	Male	No	43.0	Yes	Yes	No	T10–11	No	Yes	250	165	13
10	66	Male	No	40.7	Yes	No	No	T10–11, T11–12	No	Yes	1000	214	14
11	59	Male	No	32.9	Yes	Yes	No	T10–11	No	Yes	75	113	3
12	51	Female	No	29.5	No	Yes	No	T10–11	No	Yes	200	146	4
13	70	Male	Yes	22.8	Yes	No	No	T11–12	No	Yes	100	129	23
14	38	Male	No	32.9	Yes	No	No	T5–6	No	Yes	300	192	15
15	76	Female	No	33.6	Yes	Yes	No	T11–12, T12–L1	No	Yes	150	226	7

Abbreviations: Arthro., interbody arthrodesis; BMI, body mass index; Cal., calcified disc; EBL, estimated blood loss; LOS, total length of stay; Myel., myelopathy; ORT, operative time; Rad., radicular pain; Trans., transpleural.

Table 1.
Cases demographic, clinical and surgical data.

Case no.	Preoperative	Postoperative
1	3	3
2	2	3
3	3	7
4	3	3
5	3	4
6	3	3
7	4	5
8	6	7
9	2	3
10	3	6
11	5	7
12	N/A	N/A
13	2	3
14	2	3
15	2	2

N/A, not applicable because the patient had radiculopathy without myelopathy.

Table 2.
Motor dysfunction score of the lower extremities by the modified Japanese Orthopedic association scale.

	No.	Sex (% female)	Age	BMI	Myel. (%)	Rad. (%)	Cal. (%)	EBL (ml)	ORT (min)	LOS (days)	Trans. (%)	Chest tube (%)	Myel. stable or improved (%)
Present study	15	27	55.8	33.8	93.3	40	13.3	400	188	8	13	0	100
Bartels et al. [3]	21	57	58.8	N/A	100	4.7	100	732	222	N/A	100	100	100
Deviren et al. [4]	12	67	53	N/A	66.7	0	N/A	440	210	5	100	100	100
Kasliwal and Deutsch [5]	7	42.9	52	N/A	100	57.1	N/A	180	N/A	2.6	0	0	42.8
Malham et al. [6]	3	33	61.7	28.6	33.3	33.3	0	<50	N/A	5	66	33	100
Nacar et al. [7]	33	54	52.9	31	69.7	93.9	57.5	300	174	5	76	76	91
Uribe et al. [9]	60	47	57.9	31	70	51.6	33	290	182	5	75	22	83.3

Age, BMI, EBL, ORT, LOS values are means. Abbreviations: BMI, body mass index; Cal., calcified disc; EBL, estimated blood loss; LOS, length of stay; Myel., myelopathy; No., number of cases; N/A, not available; ORT, operative time; Rad., radicular pain; Trans., transpleural.

Table 3.
Literature review on mini-open lateral approach for symptomatic thoracic or upper lumbar disc disease: Demographic, clinical and surgical data.

3.3 Operative complication

The most frequent reported complication in the literature was intra-operative cerebrospinal fluid leak (**Table 6**). This complication was associated with calcified

	Static cage (%)	Expandable cage (%)	Autograft only (%)	Allograft only (%)	Autograft and allograft (%)	rhBMP-2 (%)	Sup. anterior inst. (%)	Sup. posterior decom. and inst. (%)	Sup. posterior decom. Only (%)
Present study	0	93	13	0	80	0	7	0	0
Bartels et al. [3]	0	0	0	0	0	0	14	0	0
Deviren et al. [4]	100	0	100	0	0	3	100	8	8
Kasliwal and Deutsch [5]	0	0	0	0	0	0	0	0	0
Malham et al. [6]	100	0	0	100	0	100	0	0	0
Nacar et al. [7]	100	0	N/A	N/A	N/A	N/A	100	3	9
Uribe et al. [9]	90	0	57	0	40	3	33	10	3

Abbreviations: Decom. = Decompression, Inst. = Instrumentation, N/A = not available, Sup. = Supplemental

Table 4.
Literature review on mini-open lateral approach for symptomatic thoracic or upper lumbar disc disease: Interbody arthrodesis and supplemental surgical data.

Level	Present study	Bartels et al. [3]	Deviren et al. [4]	Kasliwal and Deutsch [5]	Malham et al. [6]	Nacar et al. [7]	Uribe et al. [9]
T4–5	0	0	0	0	0	0	2
T5–6	1	1	0	0	0	2	1
T6–7	0	3	1	1	1	3	8
T7–8	1	2	1	2	0	8	12
T8–9	0	1	1	2	0	3	12
T9–10	2	3	0	2	1	2	8
T10–11	6	4	1	1	0	5	9
T11–12	4	8	4	0	0	8	14
T12-L1	2	0	4	0	1	6	7
L1–2	0	0	0	0	0	0	1
L2–3	0	0	0	0	0	0	1

Table 5.
Literature review on mini-open lateral approach for symptomatic thoracic or upper lumbar disc disease: Spinal levels treated.

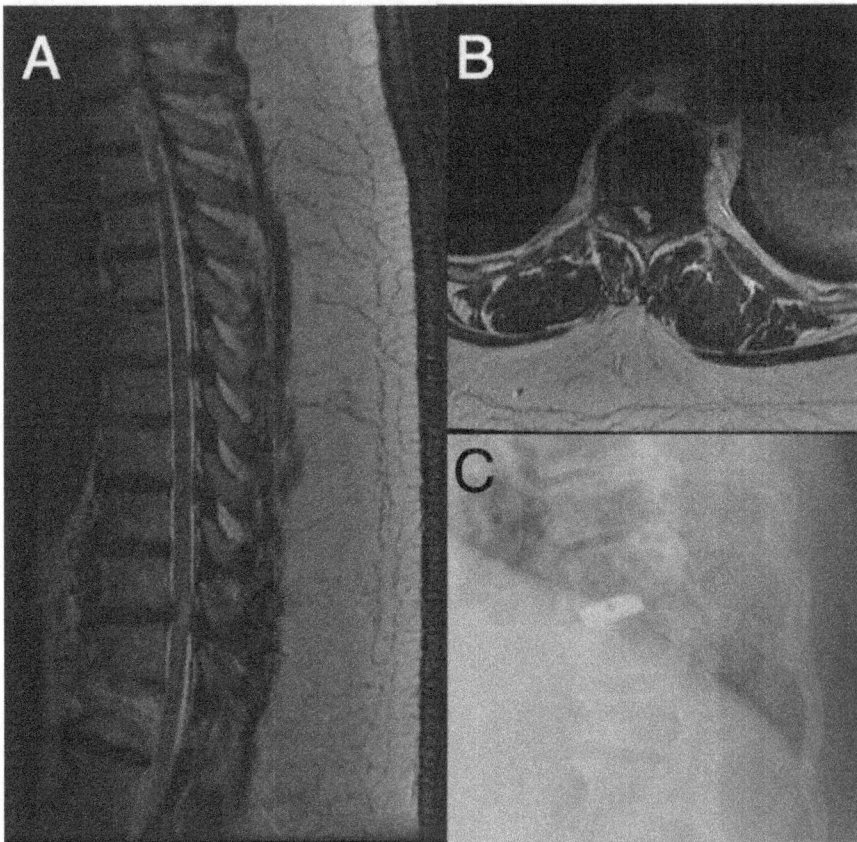

Figure 8.
Preoperative sagittal (A) and axial (B) T2-weighted magnetic resonance images of a soft disc herniation at T10–11 in a 42 years old male with body mass index of 43.0. C: Postoperative sagittal x-rays showing decompression and placement of an expandable interbody cage in the same patient.

	Present study	Bartels et al. [3]	Deviren et al. [4]	Kasliwal and Deutsch [5]	Malham et al. [6]	Nacar et al. [7]	Uribe et al. [9]
Intra-operative CSF leak	1	2	0	0	0	2	7
New lower extremity weakness	0	1	0	0	0	0	1
Neuropathic pain at incision	2	0	1	0	1	1	1
Pleural effusion	6	N/A	1	0	N/A	2	1
Pneumothorax	0	0	0	0	0	0	1
Post-op chest tube	2	N/A	1	0	N/A	2	1
Reoperation	1	0	0	0	0	0	3
Cage subsidence	2	N/A	N/A	N/A	N/A	N/A	N/A
Pseudoarthorosis	1	N/A	N/A	N/A	N/A	0	0

Abbreviation: CSF, cerebrospinal fluid; N/A, not available.

Table 6.
Literature review on mini-open lateral approach for symptomatic thoracic or upper lumbar disc disease: Complications.

disc herniations and could be successfully repaired [7, 9]. Case no. 1 who had a calcified thoracic disc herniation had a small intraoperative cerebrospinal fluid leak repaired with onlay allograft and DuraSeal® (Covidien, Waltham, MA, USA). Other postoperative complications included 6 pleural effusions, two of which required interventional radiology placement of chest tube. Costovertebral neuralgia is usually treated with neuropathic pain medication such as gabapentin or pregabalin. Topical lidocaine can also be used.

3.4 Limitations

The results of this study need to be interpreted with caution because of its retrospective nature and the limited number of cases reported. Although the outcomes were consistent with the literature, long-term follow-up would be necessary to better assess the risk of pseudoarthrosis and the persistence of resolution of symptoms.

4. Conclusion

A larger number of case series have reported successful treatment of symptomatic TDH using the mini-open lateral technique. With a short length of stay for elective cases, a relatively low complication rate and improvement of motor function in the majority of patients, the mini-open lateral approach can be considered a safe and effective procedure for symptomatic TDH. Arthrodesis using expandable cages without additional anterior instrumentation can provide satisfactory short-term outcomes. However supplemental anterior or posterior fixation should also be considered when significant pre-existing instability is suspected, when multiple contiguous levels are treated or when significant cage subsidence is noted during cage expansion.

Author details

Edna E. Gouveia[1], Mansour Mathkour[1,2], Erin McCormack[1,2], Jonathan Riffle[1,2], Olawale A. Sulaiman[1,2] and Daniel J. Denis[1,2*]

1 Department of Neurosurgery, Ochsner Clinic Foundation, New Orleans, LA, USA

2 Department of Neurosurgery, Tulane Medical Center, New Orleans, LA, USA

*Address all correspondence to: danieldenisjr@gmail.com

IntechOpen

References

[1] Han S, Jang IT. Prevalence and Distribution of Incidental Thoracic Disc Herniation, and Thoracic Hypertrophied Ligamentum Flavum in Patients with Back or Leg Pain: A Magnetic Resonance Imaging-Based Cross-Sectional Study. World Neurosurg. 2018;120:e517-ee24.

[2] Anand N, Regan JJ. Video-assisted thoracoscopic surgery for thoracic disc disease: Classification and outcome study of 100 consecutive cases with a 2-year minimum follow-up period. Spine (Phila Pa 1976). 2002;27(8):871-879.

[3] Bartels RH, Peul WC. Mini-thoracotomy or thoracoscopic treatment for medially located thoracic herniated disc? Spine (Phila Pa 1976). 2007;32 (20):E581-E584.

[4] Deviren V, Kuelling FA, Poulter G, Pekmezci M. Minimal invasive anterolateral transthoracic transpleural approach: a novel technique for thoracic disc herniation. A review of the literature, description of a new surgical technique and experience with first 12 consecutive patients. J Spinal Disord Tech. 2011;24(5):E40-E48.

[5] Kasliwal MK, Deutsch H. Minimally invasive retropleural approach for central thoracic disc herniation. Minim Invasive Neurosurg. 2011;54(4):167-171.

[6] Malham GM, Parker RM. Treatment of symptomatic thoracic disc herniations with lateral interbody fusion. J Spine Surg. 2015;1(1):86-93.

[7] Nacar OA, Ulu MO, Pekmezci M, Deviren V. Surgical treatment of thoracic disc disease via minimally invasive lateral transthoracic trans/retropleural approach: analysis of 33 patients. Neurosurg Rev. 2013;36(3): 455-465.

[8] Russo A, Balamurali G, Nowicki R, Boszczyk BM. Anterior thoracic foraminotomy through mini-thoracotomy for the treatment of giant thoracic disc herniations. Eur Spine J. 2012;21 Suppl 2:S212-S220.

[9] Uribe JS, Smith WD, Pimenta L, Hartl R, Dakwar E, Modhia UM, et al. Minimally invasive lateral approach for symptomatic thoracic disc herniation: initial multicenter clinical experience. J Neurosurg Spine. 2012;16(3):264-279.

[10] Ozgur BM, Aryan HE, Pimenta L, Taylor WR. Extreme Lateral Interbody Fusion (XLIF): a novel surgical technique for anterior lumbar interbody fusion. Spine J. 2006;6(4):435-443.

[11] Lee SY, Kim W, Lee SU, Choi KH. Relationship Between Obesity and Lumbar Spine Degeneration: A Cross-Sectional Study from the Fifth Korean National Health and Nutrition Examination Survey, 2010-2012. Metab Syndr Relat Disord. 2018.

[12] Sheng B, Feng C, Zhang D, Spitler H, Shi L. Associations between Obesity and Spinal Diseases: A Medical Expenditure Panel Study Analysis. Int J Environ Res Public Health. 2017;14(2).

[13] Oppenlander ME, Clark JC, Kalyvas J, Dickman CA. Indications and Techniques for Spinal Instrumentation in Thoracic Disk Surgery. Clin Spine Surg. 2016;29(2):E99-E106.

[14] Yue B, Chen B, Zou YW, Xi YM, Ren XF, Xiang HF, et al. Thoracic intervertebral disc calcification and herniation in adults: a report of two cases. Eur Spine J. 2016;25 Suppl 1: 118-123.

[15] Brauge D, Horodyckid C, Arrighi M, Reina V, Eap C, Mireau E, et al. Management of Giant Thoracic Disc Herniation by Thoracoscopic Approach: Experience of 53 Cases. Oper Neurosurg (Hagerstown). 2018.

[16] Cornips EM, Janssen ML, Beuls EA.
Thoracic disc herniation and acute
myelopathy: clinical presentation,
neuroimaging findings, surgical
considerations, and outcome. J
Neurosurg Spine. 2011;14(4):520-528.

[17] Gonzalez-Blohm SA, Doulgeris JJ,
Aghayev K, Lee WE, 3rd, Volkov A,
Vrionis FD. Biomechanical analysis of
an interspinous fusion device as a stand-
alone and as supplemental fixation to
posterior expandable interbody cages in
the lumbar spine. J Neurosurg Spine.
2014;20(2):209-219.

[18] Kim C, Harris JA, Muzumdar A,
Khalil S, Sclafani JA, Raiszadeh K, et al.
The effect of anterior longitudinal
ligament resection on lordosis
correction during minimally invasive
lateral lumbar interbody fusion:
Biomechanical and radiographic
feasibility of an integrated spacer/plate
interbody reconstruction device. Clin
Biomech (Bristol, Avon). 2017;43:
102-108.

Section 3

Minimally Invasive Lumbar Approaches

Minimally Invasive Laminectomy for Lumbar Stenosis with Case Series of Patients with Multi-level (3 or More Levels) Stenosis

Mick Perez-Cruet, Ramiro Pérez de la Torre and Siddharth Ramanathan

Abstract

Lumbar stenosis is the most common pathology seen and treated by spine surgeons. It is often seen in the elderly population who frequently have multiple medical co-morbidities. Traditional approaches remove the spinous process and detach paraspinous muscles to achieve adequate canal decompression. This approach can damage the posterior tension band leading to permanent muscle damage, scar tissue formation, iatrogenic flatback syndrome, and increase risk of adjacent segment disease requiring reoperation. Performing lumbar laminectomy in a cost-effective manner is critical in effectively treating patients with lumbar stenosis. This chapter reviews a minimally invasive muscle-sparing approach to treating lumbar stenosis. The technique is performed through a tubular retractor. Direct decompression of the spinal stenosis is achieved while preserving the paraspinous muscle attachments and spinous process. This technique has multiple advantages and can potentially reduce load stress on adjacent levels and subsequent adjacent level pathology leading to further surgical intervention. In addition, the procedure shows how facet fusion is performed using the patient's own locally harvested drilled morselized autograph to achieve bilateral facet fusion. By fusing the facets, we have shown that restenosis at the operative level is less likely to occur. This chapter will review a case series of multilevel lumbar stenosis including clinical outcomes.

Keywords: Lumbar stenosis, minimally invasive laminectomy, multilevel stenosis, muscle and bone preservation, autograph posterolateral fusion

1. Introduction

Over the last two decades, minimally invasive spine surgery has undergone a paradigm shift with some procedures garnering increasing favor from the neurosurgical community [1–3]. Outcomes research and an emphasis on improving intra- and post-operative outcomes have increased the importance of selecting techniques that maximize these parameters. The minimally invasive laminectomy for the treatment of spinal stenosis is one such procedure that has gained considerable momentum [2]. Several indications exist for this procedure including

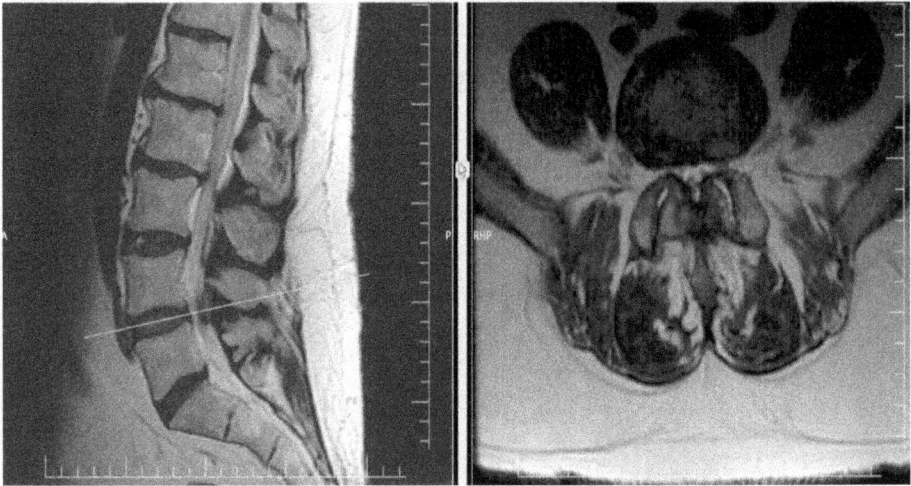

Figure 1.
A. Sagittal and B. Axial T2 weighted MRI image at the L4-5 level (marked with the green line) showing spinal stenosis caused by hypertrophy of the facets and ligamentum flavum.

primary or secondary lumbar spinal stenosis. The former is the most frequently diagnosed spinal disorder in the elderly and is a major cause of disability in this population [4].

Lumbar spinal stenosis is defined as a reduced cross-sectional diameter of the vertebral canal, usually resulting in compression of neural structures (**Figure 1**).

There are three types of compression: compression in the central portion of the spinal canal (central stenosis); in the lateral recesses of the canal (lateral recess stenosis); or a combination of stenosis in both regions. Spinal stenosis may be congenital or acquired. Congenital stenosis consists of a group of spine deformities that often present in patients diagnosed with hereditary syndromes (i.e., Achondroplasia). Symptoms of congenital stenosis typically present at a younger age than those of acquired spinal stenosis. Secondary lumbar stenosis presents with a myriad of pathological changes including hypertrophy of the ligamentum flavum, and degeneration of the facet and disc structures [5]. The compression of the central canal often leads to debilitating back pain, radiculopathy, and symptoms of neurogenic claudication, making acquired spinal stenosis one of the most critical factors in the decision for surgical intervention [6]. Lumbar canal stenosis may itself arise as a long-term consequence of sagittal balance abnormalities, spondylo-listhesis, and/or degenerative conditions.

2. Surgical techniques

There have been multiple surgical techniques developed to decompress the lumbar spine in patients suffering from lumbar stenosis. The oldest technique is the open lumbar laminectomy, which involves the removal of spinous processes, both laminae and a partial facetectomy. In performing a decompressive laminectomy, the competing forces of adequately decompressing the spine and preventing adjacent segment disease must be balanced. Adjacent segment disease describes the constellation of findings that develop as a result of pathological load forces placed on the spine. The resulting focal tissue hypertrophy and adjacent level stenosis may require additional surgical intervention (**Figure 2**).

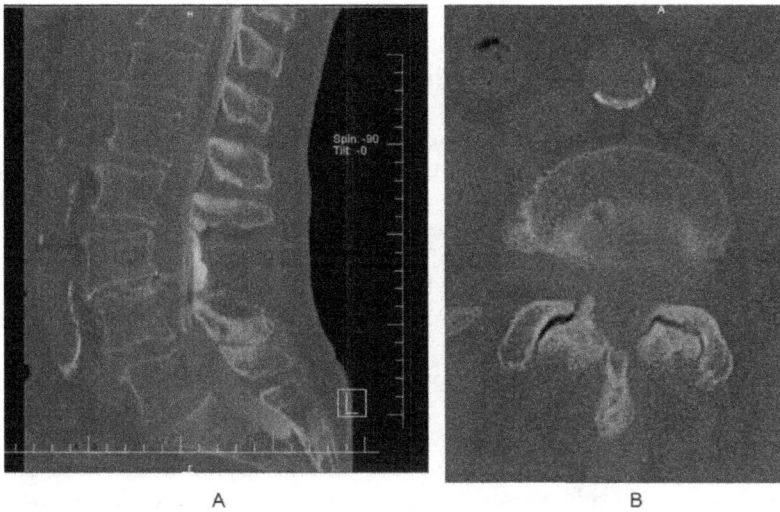

Figure 2.
A. Sagittal and B. Axial CT myelogram showing traditional laminectomy previously performed with removal of spinous processes and subsequent development of complete myelographic block at the adjacent L4-5 level requiring additional surgical intervention.

Efforts to preserve midline posterior structures have led to the introduction of minimally invasive techniques to treat degenerative lumbar stenosis. Minimally invasive spine techniques were developed to preserve the normal anatomical integrity of the spine [1, 7–9]. Fessler et al., are credited with developing the currently used technique for performing a minimally invasive laminectomy in the treatment of lumbar stenosis that will be described in this chapter [9]. Over the last several years, various improvements in microscopic visualization techniques [10] have greatly influenced surgical options. These advancements have made it feasible to utilize a unilateral laminectomy to extend instruments to the contralateral side and fully decompress the canal without the long-term spinal instability and risk for additional surgical intervention associated with traditional open procedures.

Minimally invasive laminectomy outcomes studies have confirmed its benefits [1], in patients with and without spondylolisthesis [8]. Several comparative studies have addressed minimally invasive laminectomy vs open laminectomy [11, 12], bilateral decompressive laminectomy vs muscle-sparing interlaminar approach [13], and patient outcomes based on a variety of critical analyses [5, 14, 15]. Further evolution in surgical techniques and technology aims to facilitate the minimally invasive approach [16].

3. Indications/contraindications

3.1 Patient selection

Patients presenting with lumbar stenosis may present with bilateral or unilateral leg pain, weakness, numbness, and/or paresthesias [11]. Many patients suffer from neurogenic claudication, a typical complaint where back or leg pain is aggravated by standing and walking and relieved by sitting, flexing the spine, or lying down. Symptomatic relief with lumbar flexion is often a reliable clinical sign that helps to distinguish neurogenic spinal claudication from vascular claudication. The bicycle test, in which the patient leans forward while riding a stationary bike, can also help to distinguish the two conditions. The neurological examination can be non-contributory until very late stages of the disease when a fixed motor or sensory deficits become evident. Also important in these patients is the varying degrees of walking impairment progressing over months or years [17]. Sphincter disturbance is a rare, late symptom of this condition and is usually associated with severe compression of the cauda equina, which is sometimes the result of an acute disc herniation superimposed on preexisting spinal stenosis. There are also some classical syndromic descriptions such as footdrop and acute radiculopathy. At some point, the physical examination must be able to rule out hip pathology and sacroiliac joint involvement. Multiple examinations such as Patrick Test, Faber Test, distraction, thigh thrust, compression, and Gaenslen's test are important to make these distinctions [18].

With an increasing incidence of lumbar stenosis, proper patient selection is paramount to achieving good clinical outcomes. Reoperation cases are relatively cumbersome and impose a significant burden on the patient and surgeon. As such reoperations should not be attempted until the spine surgeon has gained considerable experience with minimally invasive laminectomy approaches. In some other conditions, such as morbid obesity, there is an increased working distance from the skin to the spine, thereby increasing the technical difficulty for the surgeon. These cases are best deferred until a high level of experience and comfort with operating through a tubular retractor are achieved.

4. Radiographic work-up

The imaging workup for spinal stenosis usually begins with anteroposterior, lateral, and flexion/extension plain film X-rays, which often reveal degeneration of the anatomic structures manifesting as loss of disc space height, narrowed neural foramina, and hypertrophy of the facet joints. In some patients, dynamic films can potentially reveal instability. Magnetic resonance imaging (MRI) is the study of choice to provide diagnostic images with specific details regarding structure, dimensions, and deformities. Typical findings include degenerative disc disease, ligamentous and facet hypertrophy, and a triangularly shaped "trefoil" spinal canal. The computer tomography myelogram (CT myelogram) study can be particularly useful in patients with degenerative scoliosis, multilevel stenosis, or in cases where prior surgical intervention with instrumentation was performed. In these scenarios, the CT myelogram allows adequate visualization of the stenotic level.

5. Electromyographic studies

Some spinal stenosis patients present with a variety of clinical signs including single or multilevel compression. In those cases, the advantage of requesting additional electrophysiological studies lies in the possibility of confirming compression of individual nerve roots for surgical procedure planning [19].

6. Operative set-up and instrumentation

The minimally invasive lumbar laminectomy is performed in a standard operating room with routinely available equipment. Lateral fluoroscopy is used for confirmation of the correct surgical level. The patient is typically positioned on a Jackson table which allows normal lumbar lordosis and limits abdominal pressure to reduce surgical bleeding.

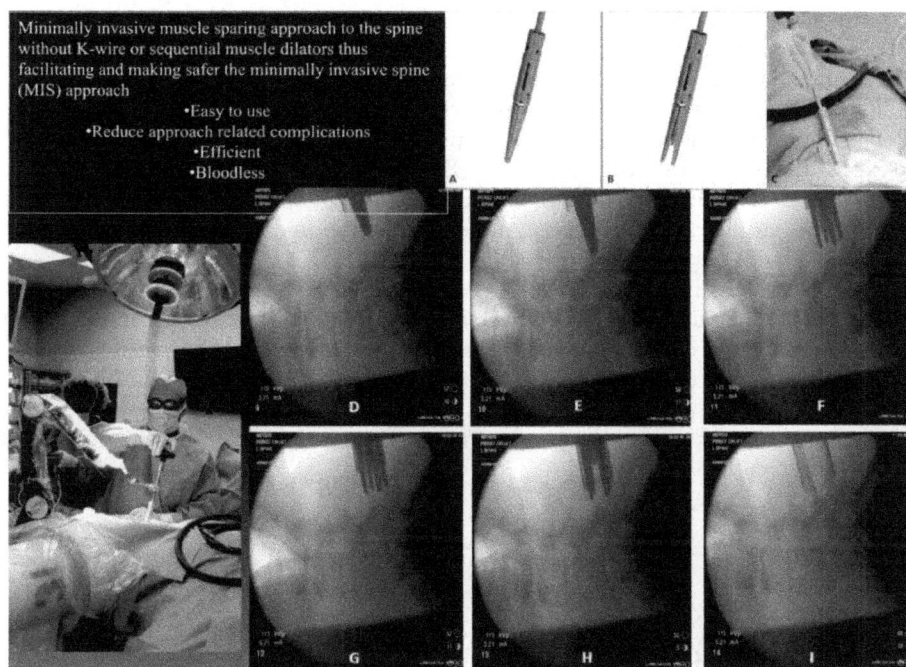

Figure 3.
The One-Step-Dilator (Thompson MIS, Salem, NH) has been developed to eliminate the need for guidewire and subsequent muscle dilators. This system allows for a bloodless, muscle-sparing approach to the spine. A., Images of One-Step-Dilator closed and B., expanded to dilate apart muscle tissue. C., Intra-operative image D–E., with fluoroscopic guided approach to the spine by gentle clockwise rotation, F., counterclockwise opening of retractor once on spine, G–H., passing of tubular retractor over dilator, I., and tubular retractor in place for performing the procedure.

7. Incision

The midline of the spine is palpated and marked. Typically, the skin incision is made a fingerbreadth lateral to the midline if one level is decompressed and no instrumentation is needed. However, for multilevel decompression, percutaneous pedicle screws are often utilized to promote fusion. When pedicle screws are required, the incision is made 3 cm lateral to the midline at the level of stenosis. This allows for adequate access to the canal for decompression and facilitates percutaneous pedicle screw placement. Once the incision is made parallel to the spinous processes, the One-Step-Dilator (Thompson MIS, Salem, NH) is used to approach the spine in a muscle-splitting fashion (**Figure 3**).

8. Laminectomy

The soft tissue on the lamina/facet surface is then removed with monopolar Bovie cautery to the sagittal extent of the tubular retractor. The caudal and rostral edges of the lamina and medial aspects of the facet are exposed. A cutting M8 match-stick burr is used to perform the ipsilateral laminectomy to expose the thickened ligamentum flavum. All drilled bone is collected using the Thompson MIS BoneBac Press, which provides excellent morselized autograft thereafter used to perform a bilateral facet fusion once adequate decompression has been completed. The benefits of morselized autograft bone material include excellent handling characteristics, adequate softness for remodeling, cost savings, and increased fusion rates [20].

The illustrations below show the steps taken to perform a minimally invasive laminectomy for stenosis. Step one, ipsilateral laminectomy shown in **Figure 4a–d**. Step two, tilt the patient slightly away from the surgeon and wand tubular retractor to expose the base of the spinous process (**Figure 4e**). The spinous process, as well as contralateral lamina, are then undercut with the high-speed burr. The contralateral lamina is undercut to the facet complex. Preservation of the ligament flavum helps protect the dura (**Figure 4f–h**).

Once bony decompression is completed, the ipsilateral ligamentum flavum is removed with an up-biting Kerrison punch. Subsequently, the contralateral ligamentum flavum can be removed. To facilitate the removal of the contralateral ligament flavum, particularly in cases of severe hypertrophy, we used a CO_2 laser to facilitate removal along with Kerrison punch, typically number 2 size. In this manner, durotomies are extremely uncommon (**Figure 5**).

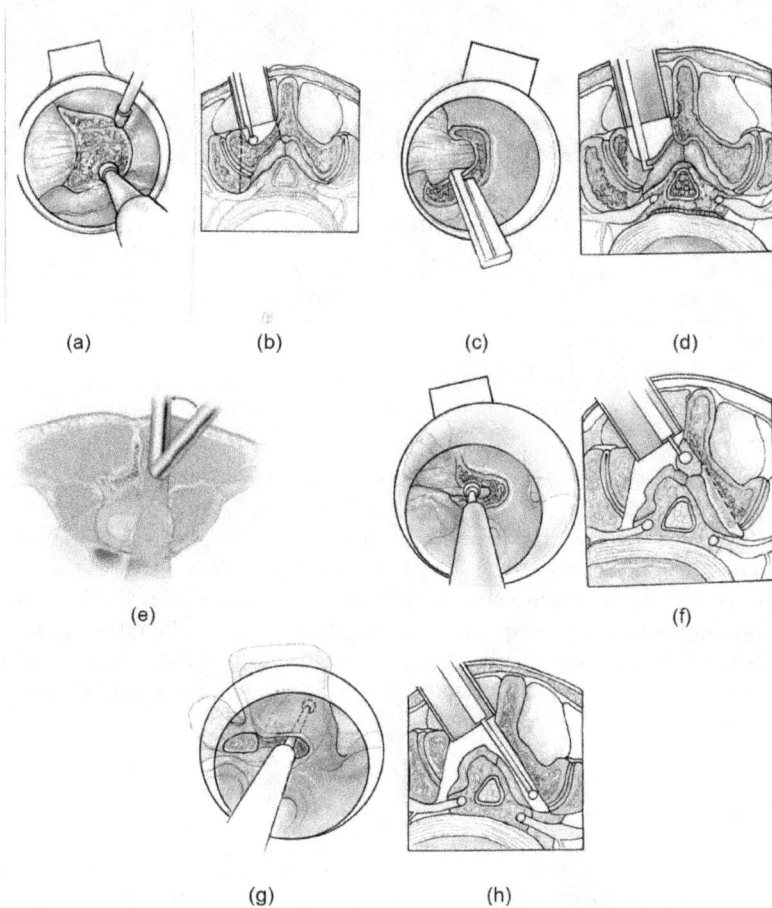

(a) (b) (c) (d)

(e) (f)

(g) (h)

Figure 4.
Illustrations showing a–d, ipsilateral laminectomy with exposure of ligamentum flavum. e, Tilting the table away from the surgeon to perform the contralateral decompression. e–h, undercutting the spinous process and contralateral lamina to achieve bony decompression. (From, An Anatomical Approach to Minimally Invasive Spine Surgery, 2nd edition. Editors MJ Perez-Cruet, RG Fessler, MY Wang, Thieme Publishing Inc, New York, New York, 2019).

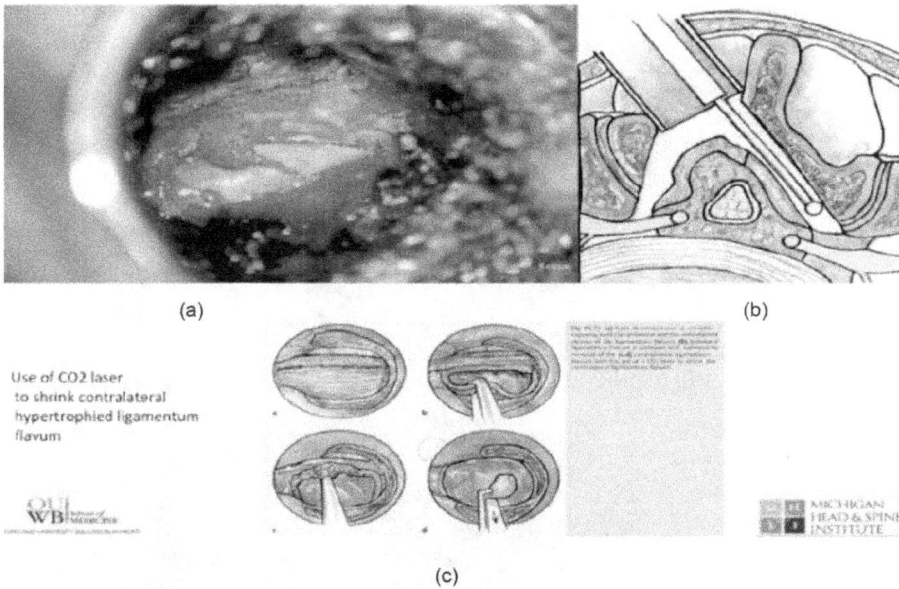

Figure 5.
a. Intraoperative photo showing dura after b. Bone decompression is performed by undercutting the spinous process and contralateral lamina with ipsilateral ligamentum flavum removed. c. Steps in removal of the hypertrophied ligamentum flavum include removal of ipsilateral ligamentum flavum followed by removal of the contralateral ligamentum flavum. This can help to reduce the risk of inadvertent durotomies. Removal of the contralateral ligamentum flavum can be aided by the use of a CO_2 laser which shrinks the contralateral ligamentum flavum making it easier to remove with a Kerrison punch. (Illustrations from, An Anatomical Approach to Minimally Invasive Spine Surgery, 2nd edition. Editors MJ Perez-Cruet, RG Fessler, MY Wang, Thieme Publishing Inc, New York, New York, 2019).

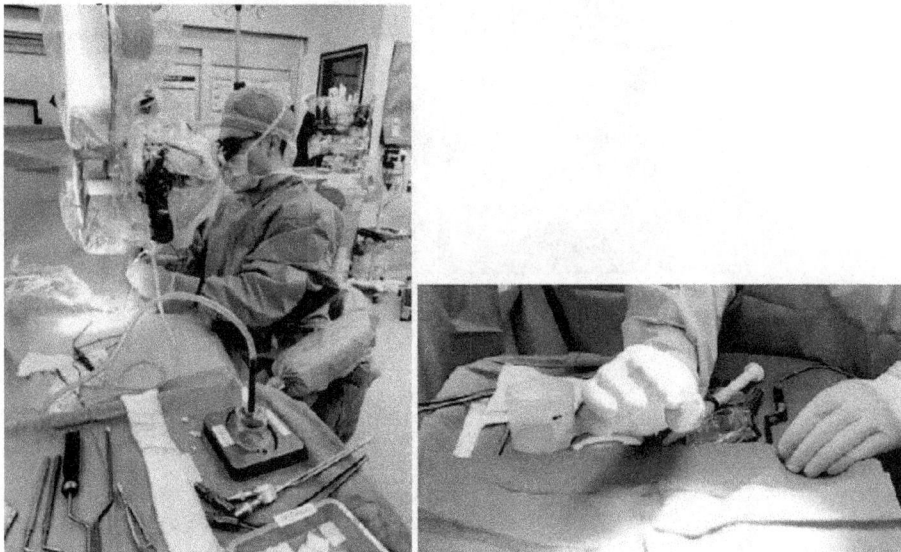

Figure 6.
Intraoperative photograph showing surgeon performing bony decompression with a drill (Stryker TPS, Kalamazoo, MI) using an M8 cutting burr and the collected B. morselized autograft using the BoneBac Press (BoneBac, Salem, NH)

The morselized autograft collected using the BoneBac press is used with no additional bone graft material needed (**Figure 6**). In-situ fusion of the bilateral decorticated facets is performed to reduce restenosis of the decompressed segment (**Figure 7**).

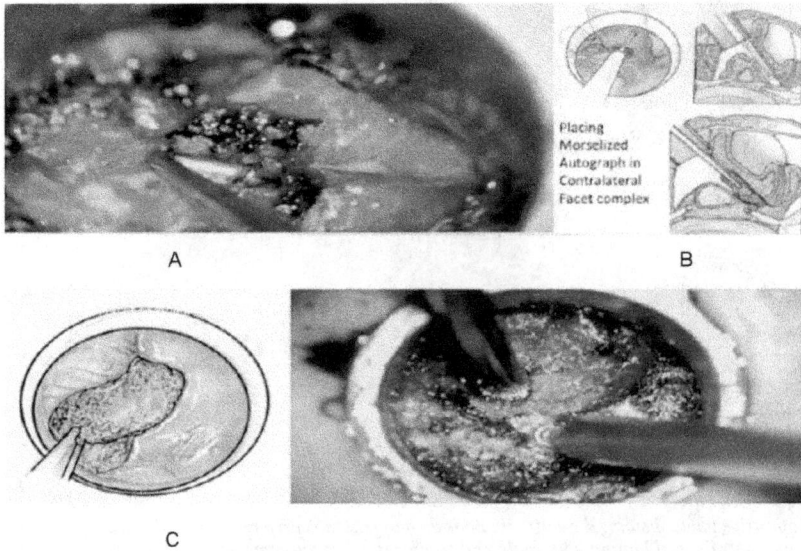

Figure 7.
A. Intraoperative photo and B. Illustration showing decortication of the contralateral facet and placement of morselized autograft into the facet complexes bilaterally. C. Illustration and intraoperative photo showing decortication of the ipsilateral facet and placement of surgical site morselized autograft.

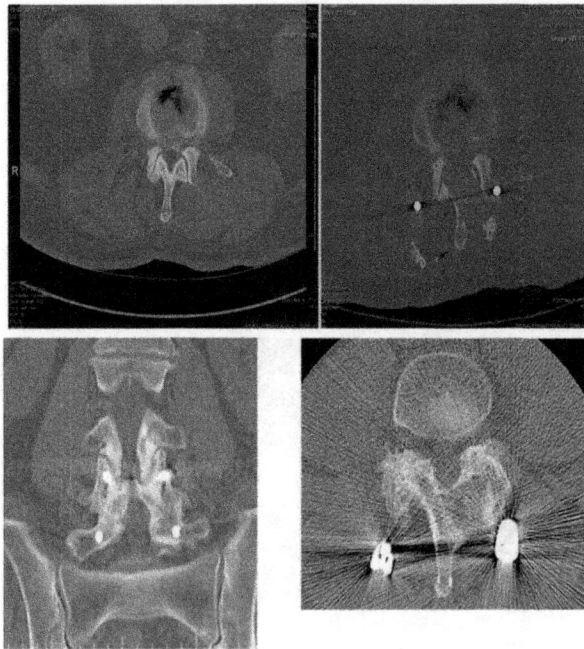

Figure 8.
Preoperative CT myelogram showing lumbar stenosis. B. Post-operative CT showing decompression by performing ipsilateral laminectomy followed by undercutting the spinous process and contralateral lamina. C. Six-month postoperative coronal and D. Axial CT showing facet fusion and maintenance of spinal canal diameter.

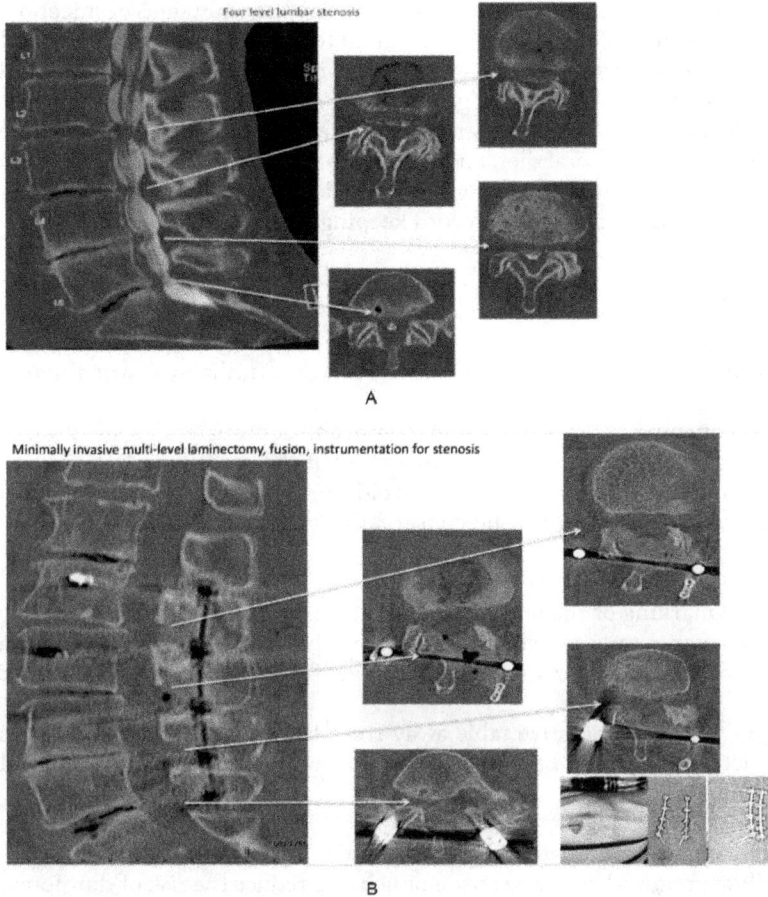

Figure 9.
Illustrative case of patient who presented with neurogenic claudication from four-level lumbar stenosis. a. Sagittal and corresponding axial MRI showing lumbar stenosis at L2-3, L3-L4, L4-L5, and L5-S1 levels. b. Post-operative sagittal and corresponding axial CT showing decompression at each level with postoperative incisions and anteroposterior and lateral x-rays. Note adequate central canal decompression with preservation of the spinous processes.

In cases of scoliotic deformity of spondylolisthesis (**Figure 8**) or multilevel decompression, (**Figure 9**) percutaneous pedicle screw instrumentation is applied to improve fusion rates.

The collected morselized autograft is then placed via the tubular retractor into the bilaterally decorticated facet complexes to achieve a bilateral posterior facet fusion. Facet fusion reduces the rates of restenosis by stabilizing the segment (**Figure 8**).

With complete hemostasis, the fascia is reapproximated with 2-0 vicryl suture, followed by multilayer subcutaneous closure. Final skin closure is accomplished with the application of Prineo adhesive dressing and Dermabond (Johnson & Johnson). This avoids the need for skin staple or suture removal and leaves a cosmetically pleasing scar.

9. Post-operative care

Post-operatively, the patient is transferred to the floor for recovery. Drainage, if utilized, can usually be removed within 24 hours. Patients are counseled regarding proper wound care and instructed to return if they have any signs of infection or deterioration in neurological status. The initial follow-up visit is most often scheduled for 2 weeks after surgery and at 3 and 6 months post-operatively. Physical therapy is also initiated as needed, generally beginning 2 weeks after surgery. Most individuals can be sent home the same day of the procedure when they are freely ambulating, tolerate an oral diet, and are able to void spontaneously. Standard information, including universal signs of infection, is conveyed in a regularized form for patient information and record keeping.

10. Complication avoidance

- Confirmation of the correct surgical level is done utilizing C-arm fluoroscopy.

- Initial opening of the ligamentum flavum and contralateral ligamentum flavum removal is often the most difficult portion of the procedure. Delicate and careful manipulation is mandatory to avoid dural defects. If dural injuries occur, the majority of them can be conservatively treated with a Gelfoam to cover the defect.

- Proper marking of the midline and identification of relevant anatomical structures is paramount to avoid difficulties with orientation. The ligamentum flavum may be utilized to assure the surgeon of the orientation of the procedure.

- Slightly tilt the operative table away from the surgeon and wand the tubular retractor to view the base of the spinous process to perform the contralateral decompression.

- Shrinking the contralateral ligamentum flavum with a CO2 laser or CUSA can facilitate removal with a Kerrison punch and reduce the risk of durotomy.

- When working toward the contralateral side, the smooth base of the Kerrison rongeur should be kept against the dura to reduce the risk of dural laceration.

- Approach each level separately when treating patients with multi-level stenosis. This allows direct visualization and facilitates adequate decompression.

- Percutaneous pedicle screw fixation reduces the rates of recurrent spinal stenosis at the level of decompression by assuring adequate arthrodesis.

11. Clinical case series

A retrospective analysis was performed of patients undergoing 3 or more levels of minimally invasive laminectomy for lumbar stenosis as seen in **Figure 10**.

Thirty-three consecutive patients were analyzed with clinical characteristics as seen below (**Table 1**). The most common levels treated are seen in **Table 2** and medical co-morbidities are seen in **Table 3**. The average estimated blood loss was 190 cc. Surgical time averaged 3 hours. Hospital stays averaged 3-4 days. Complications rates were relatively low (**Table 4**). Visual analog score (VAS) back and leg pain and Oswestry disability index (ODI) improved as seen in **Figure 11**. These improvements were found to be statistically significant at 24-month follow-up compared with pre-operative values. One patient (3%) underwent adjacent level

Pre-operative MRI L2-3/L3-4/L4-5 stenosis

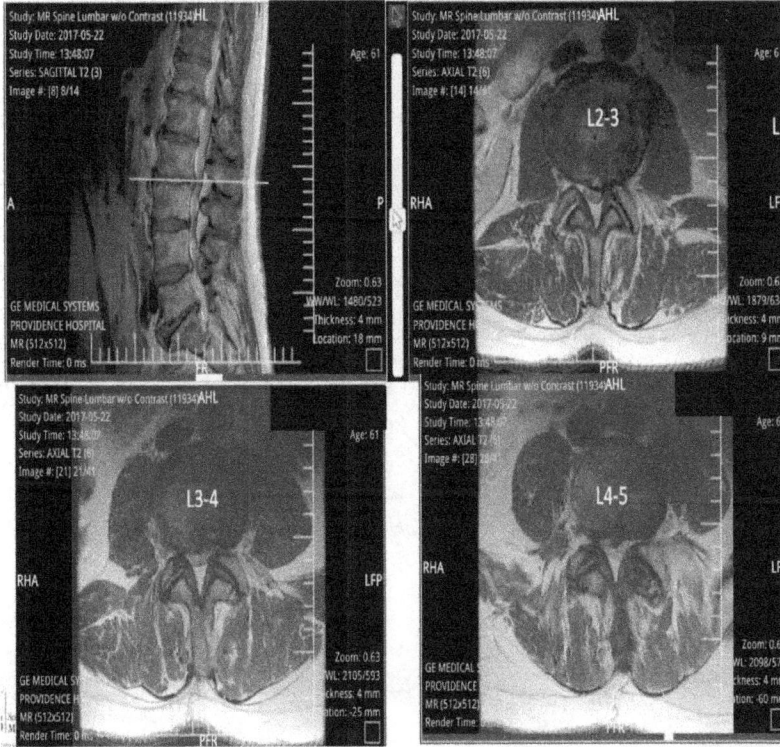

(a)

Post-op MRI after L2-3/L3-4/L4-5 MIS laminectomy: Note preservation of spinous process and paraspinous muscle anatomy

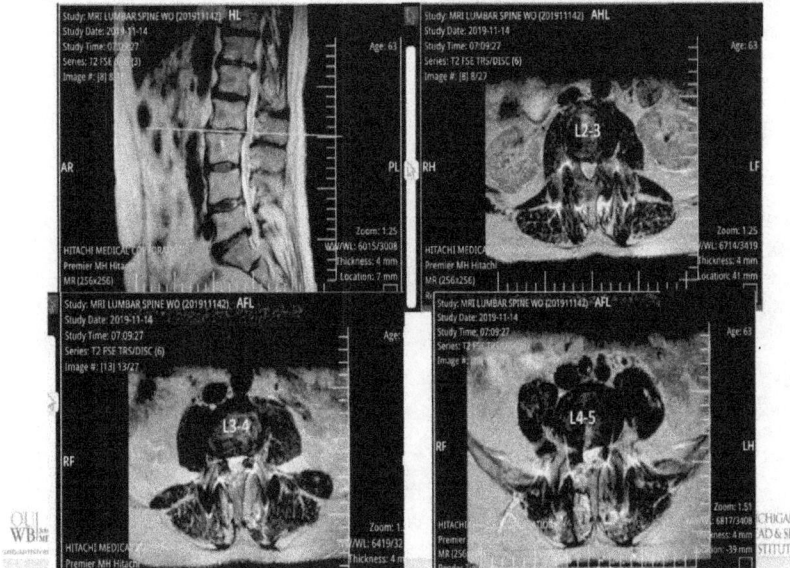

(b)

Figure 10.
Pre and post-operative T2 weighted sagittal and corresponding axial MRI images of patient who underwent L2-3/L3-4/L4-5 minimally invasive laminectomy for stenosis. Note on post-operative MRI preservation of spinous process and paraspinous muscle anatomy while achieving adequate canal decompression.

Patient characteristics (n=33)

33 patients analyzed in retrospective study
Mean follow-up of 31.7 months (minimum 15 months, maximum 48 months)
Gender distribution of 26 males, (78.78%) 7 females (21.2%)
Mean age at surgery of 70.12 years, (minimum 54, maximum 81)
Number of decompressed levels, 3 in 29 patients (87.87%), 4 in 3 patients (9.09%), 5 in 1 (3.03%)

Table 1.
Clinical characteristics of patients undergoing minimally invasive laminectomy (3 or more levels).

LEVEL OF COMPROMISE (n=33)

LEVEL OF AFFECTION	NUMBER
T10-T11	1
T12-L1	1
L1-L2	5
L2-L3	29
L3-L4	33
L4-L5	30
L5-S1	5

Table 2.
Levels treated with lumbar stenosis. Most common levels treated were L2-3, L3-4 and L4-5.

Frequency of Comorbidities (n=33)

Disease	Number of patients (n=33)
Reumatoid arthritis	15
Diabetes mellitus	12
Hypertension	7
Cancer	7
Morbid obesity (Grade III)	4
Asthma	3
Coronary artery disease	2
Chron disease	1

Table 3.
Medical co-morbidities seen in patients treated with 3 or more levels of lumbar stenosis.

Average estimated blood loss:	190.63cc
Surgical time :	3 hours
Hospital stay:	3.5 days
Immediate complications :	2 (6.6%)
Reoperation:	1
Perioperative Death:	0

Complications prolonging hospitalization	Number (n=33)
Acute urinary retention	2 (2.98%)
Postoperative ileus	2(2.98%)
Post-operative pain prolonging hosp.	1(1.4%)
Cardiac arhythmia	1(1.4%)
Atelectasis	1(1.4%)

- Postoperative complications:
- -1 case of infection managed with reoperation and antibiotic (3.3%)
- -1 Case of PO Brain infarction with no major sequelae (3.3%)

Table 4.
Operative characteristics, complication rates, and reoperations of patients undergoing multi-level (3 or more levels) minimally invasive laminectomy for stenosis. There was a relatively low rate of complications in these patients.

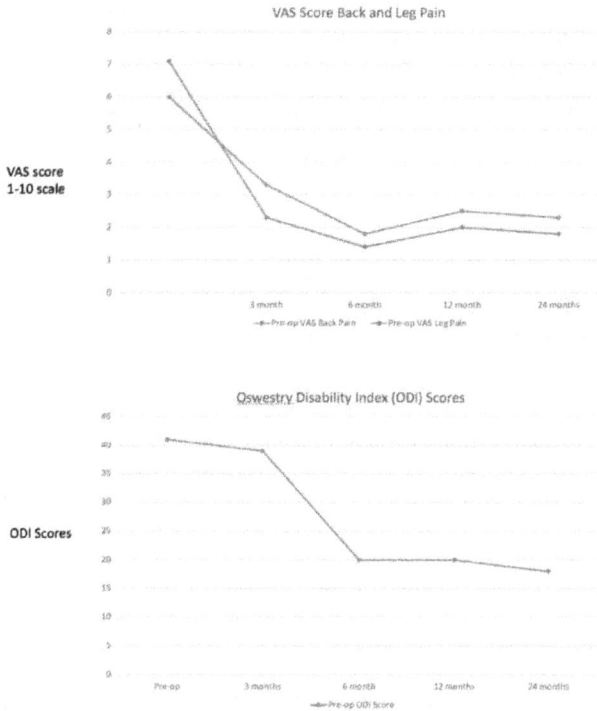

Figure 11.
Visual analogue score (VAS) back and leg pain and Oswestry disability index (ODI) improved as seen above.

laminectomy, decompression, and instrumentation for adjacent level disease. This patient had multilevel degenerative disc disease of the lumbar spine. He initially underwent a L2-3, L3-4, and L4-5 MIS laminectomy, fusion, and pedicle screw instrumentation for multi-level stenosis. He subsequently developed L5-S1 lumbar stenosis and underwent adjacent level decompression, fusion and instrumentation. He has since returned to work and has normal activities of daily living.

This series shows the benefits of minimally invasive laminectomy for stenosis. We feel that preservation of the normal anatomy (i.e., spinous process and paraspinous muscle) improves long-term outcomes, fusion rates, and complications of patients suffering from lumbar stenosis and reduce adjacent level disease requiring reoperation.

12. Conclusion

With an increased incidence of lumbar spinal stenosis and a commensurate rise in the number of operations performed to treat this condition, the minimally invasive laminectomy for lumbar stenosis represents an incredible opportunity to improve existing surgical outcomes. Completing the surgical procedure through a microscopic technique affords smaller incision, less postoperative pain, and overall quicker recovery. Additional benefits include excellent long-term outcomes and an sextremely low rate of additional surgical intervention at the operative or adjacent levels.

Potential conflict of interest

Mick Perez-Cruet COI
Thompson MIS/Bonebac: Stock ownership
Orthofix: Speaker Bureau, consultant
Thieme Publishing Inc.: Royalties

Author details

Mick Perez-Cruet[1,2*], Ramiro Pérez de la Torre[2] and Siddharth Ramanathan[1]

1 Department of Neurosurgery, Oakland University William Beaumont, School of Medicine, Rochester, MI, United States

2 Department of Neurosurgery, Michigan Head and Spine Institute, Royal Oak, MI, United States

*Address all correspondence to: perezcruet@yahoo.com

IntechOpen

References

[1] Epstein NE. Lower complication and reoperation rates for laminectomy rather than MI TLIF/other fusions for degenerative lumbar disease/ spondylolisthesis: A review. Surgical Neurology International. 2018;**9**:55. DOI: 10.4103/sni.sni_26_18

[2] Horan J, Ben Husien M, Bolger C. Bilateral laminectomy through a unilateral approach (minimally invasive) versus open laminectomy for lumbar spinal stenosis. British Journal of Neurosurgery. 2021;**35**(2):161-165. DOI: 10.1080/02688697.2020.1777253

[3] Basil GW, Wang MY. Trends in outpatient minimally invasive spine surgery. Journal of Spine Surgery. 2019;**5**(Suppl 1):S108-S114. DOI: 10.21037/jss.2019.04.17

[4] Bae HW, Rajaee SS, Kanim LE. Nationwide trends in the surgical management of lumbar spinal stenosis. Spine (Phila Pa 1976). 2013;**38**(11): 916-926. DOI: 10.1097/BRS. 0b013e3182833e7c

[5] Austevoll IM, Gjestad R, Brox JI, Solberg TK, Storheim K, Rekeland F, et al. The effectiveness of decompression alone compared with additional fusion for lumbar spinal stenosis with degenerative spondylolisthesis: a pragmatic comparative non-inferiority observational study from the Norwegian Registry for Spine Surgery. European Spine Journal. 2017;**26**(2):404-413. DOI: 10.1007/s00586-016-4683-1

[6] Kitab S, Lee BS, Benzel EC. Redefining lumbar spinal stenosis as a developmental syndrome: an MRI-based multivariate analysis of findings in 709 patients throughout the 16- to 82-year age spectrum. Journal of Neurosurgery. Spine. 2018;**29**(6):654-660. DOI: 10.3171/2018.5. SPINE18100

[7] Mobbs RJ, Li J, Sivabalan P, Raley D, Rao PJ. Outcomes after decompressive laminectomy for lumbar spinal stenosis: comparison between minimally invasive unilateral laminectomy for bilateral decompression and open laminectomy: clinical article. Journal of Neurosurgery. Spine. 2014;**21**(2):179-186. DOI: 10.3171/2014.4. SPINE13420

[8] Alimi M, Hofstetter CP, Pyo SY, Paulo D, Härtl R. Minimally invasive laminectomy for lumbar spinal stenosis in patients with and without preoperative spondylolisthesis: Clinical outcome and reoperation rates. Journal of Neurosurgery. Spine. 2015;**22**(4):339-352. DOI: 10.3171/2014.11.SPINE13597

[9] Guiot BH, Khoo LT, Fessler RG. A minimally invasive technique for decompression of the lumbar spine. Spine (Phila Pa 1976). 2002;**27**(4): 432-438. DOI: 10.1097/00007632-200202150-00021

[10] Yeung AT, Tsou PM. Posterolateral endoscopic excision for lumbar disc herniation. Surgical technique, outcome, and complications in 307 consecutive cases. Spine. 2002;**27**(7):722-731. DOI: 10.1097/00007632-200204010-00009

[11] Phan K, Mobbs R. Minimally invasive versus open laminectomy for lumbar stenosis: A systematic review and meta-analysis. Spine (Phila Pa 1976). 2016;**41**(2):E91-E100. DOI: 10.1097/BRS.0000000000001161

[12] Overdevest GM, Jacobs W, Vleggert-Lankamp C, Thomé C, Gunzburg R, Peul W. Effectiveness of posterior decompression techniques compared with conventional laminectomy for lumbar stenosis. Cochrane Database of Systematic Reviews. 2015;**3**:CD010036. DOI: 10.1002/14651858.CD010036.pub2

[13] Arai Y, Hirai T, Yoshii T, Sakai K, Kato T, Enomoto M, et al. A prospective

comparative study of 2 minimally invasive decompression procedures for lumbar spinal canal stenosis: unilateral laminectomy for bilateral decompression (ULBD) versus muscle-preserving interlaminar decompression (MILD). Spine (Phila Pa 1976). 2014;**39**(4):332-340. DOI: 10.1097/ BRS.0000000000000136

[14] Nerland US, Jakola AS, Solheim O, Weber C, Rao V, Lønne G, et al. Minimally invasive decompression versus open laminectomy for central stenosis of the lumbar spine: Pragmatic comparative effectiveness study. BMJ. 2015;**350**:h1603. DOI: 10.1136/ bmj.h1603

[15] Austevoll IM, Gjestad R, Solberg T, Storheim K, Brox JI, Hermansen E, et al. Comparative effectiveness of microdecompression alone vs decompression plus instrumented fusion in lumbar degenerative spondylolisthesis. JAMA Network Open. 2020;**3**(9):e2015015. DOI: 10.1001/ jamanetworkopen.2020.15015

[16] Elswick CM, Strong MJ, Joseph JR, Saadeh Y, Oppenlander M, Park P. Robotic-assisted spinal surgery: Current generation instrumentation and new applications. Neurosurgery Clinics of North America. 2020;**31**(1):103-110. DOI: 10.1016/j.nec.2019.08.012

[17] Bumann H, Nüesch C, Loske S, Byrnes SK, Kovacs B, Janssen R, et al. Severity of degenerative lumbar spinal stenosis affects pelvic rigidity during walking. The Spine Journal. 2020;**20**(1): 112-120. DOI: 10.1016/j.spinee.2019. 08.016

[18] Geisler FH, Heiney JP. Stabilization of the sacroiliac joint with the sacroiliac bone surgical implant. In: Perez-Cruet M, Fessler RG, Wang M, editors. An Anatomic Approach to Minimally Invasive Spine Surgery. New York, NY: Thieme Medical Publishers; 2019. pp. 416-439

[19] Zileli M, Crostelli M, Grimaldi M, Mazza O, Anania C, Fornari M, et al. Natural course and diagnosis of lumbar spinal stenosis: WFNS spine committee recommendations. World Neurosurgery X. 2020;**7**:100073. DOI: 10.1016/j.wnsx.2020.100073

[20] Zakaria HM, Mansour T, Telemi E, Xiao S, Bazydlo M, Schultz L, et al. Patient demographic and surgical factors that affect completion of patient-reported outcomes 90 days and 1 year after surgery: Analysis from the Michigan spine surgery improvement collaborative (MSSIC). Spine. World Neurosurgery. 2019;**130**:e259-e271. DOI: 10.1016/j.wneu.2019.06.058

Chapter 7

Advancements in Minimally Invasive Lateral Interbody Fusion

Ronald Sahyouni, Luis D. Diaz-Aguilar and Donald Blaskiewicz

Abstract

Extreme lateral interbody fusion (XLIF) is a popular surgical technique to address a wide variety of spinal pathologies. The purpose of this chapter is to explore the XLIF procedure, including indications for its use, post-fusion operative outcomes, intraoperative considerations, and advantages and disadvantages over similar fusion techniques.

Keywords: spinal fusion, extreme lateral interbody fusion, lateral lumbar interbody fusion, minimally invasive spine surgery, lumbar spine surgery

1. Introduction

Instrumented fusion of the spine is a proven method for treating a variety of spinal pathologies, such as deformity, instability and iatrogenic instability. Historically, instrumented fusion has been an open procedure, with various approaches to the spinal column including anterior lumbar interbody fusion (ALIF), posterior lumbar interbody fusion (PLIF), transformainal lumbar interbody fusion (TLIF), and posterior intertransverse fusion (PLF) [1–8]. However, advancements in minimally invasive surgery (MIS) have changed the landscape of instrumented spinal fusion procedures, and the focus of contemporary clinical practice emphasizes MIS fusion techniques because of their lower rate of complications, shorter recovery time, smaller incisions, and reduced intraoperative blood loss [9].

Extreme lateral interbody fusion (XLIF [NuVasive, San Diego, CA, USA]) is a novel minimally invasive technique in which the disc space is accessed laterally using a lateral transpsoatic approach [10]. The XLIF approach, which was introduced by Pimenta in 2001 and further developed in the same decade [11, 12], has been successfully shown to treat degenerative disc disease (DDD), deformity, trauma, tumor, and infection [13]. The purpose of this chapter is to explore the XLIF procedure, including indications for its use, post-fusion operative outcomes, intraoperative considerations, and advantages and disadvantages over similar fusion techniques.

2. Surgical terminology

While the MIS lateral interbody fusion technique is referred to as XLIF in this chapter, several other names exist for the same surgery. As of late, a general name for the surgery, lateral lumbar interbody fusion (LLIF), has emerged and increased in popularity within the literature [14, 15]. Similarly, comparable industry-sponsored surgical techniques have been coined, including the direct lateral interbody fusion (DLIF [Medtroinic, Memphis, TN, USA]) [15]. Although the term XLIF is chosen to described the MIS lateral interbody fusion technique in this chapter, it is important for readers to understand that the same surgical technique may be referenced with other names in the larger scope of the literature.

3. Anatomy

The XLIF approach is a retroperitoneal, transpsoas approach to the spinal column. The retroperitoneal space bordered by the posterior part of the transversalis fascia and the posterior parietal peritoneum, and encompasses critical organs including kidneys, adrenal glands, ureters, ascending, and descending segments of the colon, neurovascular structures including the aorta, inferior vena cava (IVC), lumbar plexus, and sympathetic trunk. In addition, spinal levels located in the posterior retroperitoneal space include T12 to the sacrum, and the psoas muscle is also located within this span.

Several muscular structures and layers are traversed during the XLIF procedure. First, the lateral abdominal muscle layers, starting superiorly from the external abdominal oblique, internal abdominal oblique, transversus abdominis, and rectus abdominis muscles, must be carefully dissected. Critical neurological structures to be mindful of during dissection include the iliohypogastric and ilioinguinal branches of L1, which supply sensation to skin over the lateral gluteal and hypogastric regions.

The psoas muscle, which is the major muscle encountered during the XLIF approach, acts as a hip abductor, lateral rotator, and flexor. The superficial part and origin of the psoas muscle begins at the T12 and L1 to L4 vertebrae, overlying the lumbar plexus. The deep part of the psoas muscle takes origin from the transverse processes of lumbar vertebrae L1 to L5, and the entire psoas muscle crosses the pelvic brim and inserts on the lesser trochanter of the femur. Of particular anatomical importance is the femoral nerve which is derived from the anterior rami of nerve roots, L2, L3 and L4. The femoral nerve is the largest branch of the lumbar plexus. The femoral nerve lies within the posterior 1/4th of the disc space at L4/5. Intraoperative nerve monitoring is helpful in reducing the risk of nerve injury [16, 17].

Furthermore, the diaphragm, and associated lumbar attachments of the right and left crura, pose an anatomical consideration during an XLIF procedure. Namely, adequate mobilization of the diaphragm around the thoracolumbar junction allows for improved disc exposure and a wider window through which a lateral XLIF corpectomy may be performed [18]. In addition, angled approaches may allow for successful XLIF completion with avoidance of the diaphragm.

4. Indications for XLIF

There are multiple indications for the XLIF procedure, including [19]:

- Spondylolisthesis

- Herniated Disc

- DDD

- Post-laminectomy instability

- Adjacent Segment Disease

- Degenerative Scoliosis

- Thoracic disc herniations

- Need for corpectomy for trauma or tumor

Oftentimes, the XLIF surgical approach is considered in patients with symptoms refractory to other treatments, including physical therapy, pain medication, and steroid injections. Additionally, specific spinal levels are best treated with the XLIF technique. High-risk patients with complicated histories may further benefit from XLIF surgery due to its minimally invasive nature. Minimal blood loss, tissue damage, and post-operative discomfort make it a viable option for complicated patients.

Furthermore, several patient conditions exclude the consideration of XLIF as a viable surgical technique. These conditions include, but are not limited to:

- Fusion below the pelvic brim (L5-S1), which inhibits access to the disc space from the lateral position

- Bilateral retroperitoneal scarring

- Complicated and/or high-grade spondylolisthesis

- Low riding L4-L5 space, with limited access to the disc space

- Spinal deformities resulting in significant spinal rotation

- Poor bone stock due to osteoarthritis, reducing the probability of successful vertebral fusion

5. Procedure

Following endotracheal anesthesia and intravenous line placement, the patient is positioned on their side in a true 90-degree lateral decubitus position [11]. The side through which the XLIF is performed is determined based on anatomical and clinical consideration. X-ray imaging is performed using a cross-table anterior–posterior (AP), and lateral technique to locate and confirm the disc of interest, and plan the surgical incision. The skin is aseptically treated and patient's spine is placed in flexion to achieve sufficient distance between the ribcage and iliac crest. Next, the pathway for instrumentation is calculated using a k-wire and lateral fluoroscopic imaging to identify the mid-position of the lumbar disc. This position is marked on the patient's lateral side at the level of the diseased disc and will serve as the working portal throughout the operation [11].

Prior to the introduction of surgical instruments, a second mark is made posterior to the working portal at the intersection of the erector spinae and abdominal oblique muscles. A 3–4 cm lateral incision is made here, large enough to allow the entry of the surgeon's index finger, which will be inserted anteriorly and advanced until the retroperitoneal space and peritoneum are identified [11]. Placement of the surgeon's finger will help protect the peritoneum, in which the visceral organs are encased, from injury while instruments are passed into and out of the working portal.

Next, the primary 3–4 cm incision is made at the mark of the working portal and the initial tubular dilator is introduced laterally, with the index finger guiding it towards the psoas muscle and away from neurovasculature and the peritoneal sac. Electromyography (EMG) is performed at the psoas muscle to steer clear of lumbar nerve roots and branches of the lumbar plexus. The psoas muscle is delicately parted between the middle and anterior third of the muscle, allowing for direct manipulation of the spine with minimal risk of damage to nervous structures and large vessels coursing anterior to the operative corridor. Additional tubular dilators are introduced to further increase the dimension of the working portal, throughout which nerve monitoring and X-ray imaging are continued to ensure safety and precision at the level of the damaged disc. Once the working portal is dilated to an appropriate diameter, a retractor is inserted and expanded in a cranio-caudal direction to the appropriate aperture [11]. The aperture of the retractor may be adjusted periodically during the operation on an as-needed basis to provide appropriate visualization and access to the spinal column. A light and camera may then be inserted and fusion may now begin.

At this point, discectomy is performed in a standard fashion and using standard surgical instruments. The diseased disc is removed with preservation of the posterior annulus, and the interbody implant is able to be accommodated in the space, resting on the lateral margins of the epiphyseal ring to increase end plate support [11]. To close the surgical site, the operative site is irrigated and hemostasis is achieved. The facial and subcutaneous layers are sutured closed, with some skin glue to close the most superficial layers. Depending on the individual patients' status, additional support including pedicle screws, plates, or rods may be inserted to stabilize the patient.

6. Intraoperative risks

The XLIF surgical approach has been associated with a unique set of complications involving multiple neurovascular structures and visceral organs that may be iatrogenically damaged during soft tissue dissection or surgical instrumentation.

6.1 Nerve injury

Nerve injury is among the most commonly cited complications following XLIF procedures. Recent reviews have suggested that neurological injury - specifically ipsilateral sensorimotor deficits of the groin and/or thigh - may be experienced transiently by 30–40% of patients postoperatively and permanently by 4–5% of patients [15, 20]. Structures that may be damaged during the surgical approach and instrumentation include the sympathetic chain located in the lateral aspect of vertebral body, the lumbosacral plexus containing the genitofemoral nerve located on the anterior surface of psoas muscle, and the superior hypogastric plexus.

The femoral branch of the genitofemoral nerve provides sensation to the scrotum in males, mons pubis in females, and anterior thigh in both sexes while the genital branch provides motor innervation to the cremaster muscle in males. Radiographic studies have demonstrated the close proximity of the genitofemoral nerve to the L2/L3 disc space [21] while cadaveric studies suggest anatomic variation in the course of the genitofemoral nerve in 40–50% of individuals [22]. These anatomical factors place the nerve at high risk of trauma with no zone of absolute safety during the XLIF approach [23], so surgeons must carefully navigate the surgical interval to avoid neurological injury. Furthermore, prolonged muscle retraction time over 20–40 minutes per level has been shown to greatly increase the risk of nerve injury [24], and electromyographic monitoring has been shown to reliability predict nerve dysfunction [25], highlighting the importance of reducing operative time. Newer retractor systems and more refined surgical techniques may eventually decrease the incidence of retractor-related nerve damage [26, 27].

More recent studies have also demonstrated small (1.7–4.8%) risks of femoral and obturator nerve neurapraxia and/or axonotmesis in the immediate post-operative period, though full recovery is expected within 3 months [28, 29]. Of note, femoral nerve injury is almost exclusively observed at the L4-L5 lumbar levels as anatomic studies have demonstrated that the femoral nerve lies more proximal to the ideal discectomy site at L4-L5, placing it at increased risk within that region [30, 31]. Several studies have also noted the risk of contralateral femoral nerve injury secondary to overzealous endplate removal and osteophyte distraction [32, 33].

Additional nervous structures that may be damaged intraoperatively include the ilioinguinal, iliohypogastric, and lateral femoral cutaneous nerves that course through the retroperitoneal space and lateral abdominal wall, though the literature is scarce on these complications. Retrograde ejaculation is also theoretically possible if there is damage to the superior hypogastric plexus, but there has yet to be a report of this complication following XLIF. Finally, bowel and bladder dysfunction may be a rare complication associated with lumbosacral plexus injury.

6.2 Vascular injury

Vascular injury is extremely rare in XLIFs compared to approaches such as the ALIF, as great vessels such as the aorta and iliac arteries are avoided. However, dissection of segmental arteries can result in serious complications that may occur during or shortly after an XLIF procedure. In one case, a large retroperitoneal hematoma was detected five days following an L3-L4 and L4-L5 XLIF [34]. Arteriography identified active bleeding from the L2 segmentary artery as the underlying etiology. This branch was promptly embolized with fibre coils, and the patient suffered no further complications. A similar case by Santillan et al. described the development of a retroperitoneal hematoma 48 hours after an uneventful L2-L3 XLIF [35]. An angiogram showed iatrogenic arterial wall disruption of the L2 lumbar artery and a traumatic pseudoaneurysm, both of which were successfully embolized with no further sequelae. Finally, a fatal case of bleeding was reported by Assina et al. in a 50-year old patient undergoing XLIF for an L4-L5 degenerative disc [36]. Imaging showed that the anterior detachable blade tip (Scoville type retractor) had transected the right common iliac vein and was within the lumen of the left common iliac vein. Furthermore, multiple perforations along the distal IVC were noted. Despite 29 units of packed red blood cells, multiple other heroic measures, and a 4-week intensive care unit stay, the patient developed a retroperitoneal abscess with bacteremia that ultimately led to hemodynamic instability and fatal multiple organ failure secondary to septic shock.

6.3 Visceral structures

Injury to non-neurovascular structures is uncommon in the setting of XLIFs and described primarily in case reports. The ureter traverses the retroperitoneal space close to XLIF surgical corridor in approximately 16% of cases [37] and may be damaged by retractors or retroperitoneal dissection particularly at the L2-L3 level [38], though no cases of urological injury have been reported on XLIFs specifically. However, ureteral complications have been reported in several patients undergoing OLIF, which utilizes a similar surgical approach to the XLIF [39–42].

Peritoneal damage following XLIF is exceedingly rare and has been described in just a few case reports. Balsano et al. reported an iatrogenic perforation of the splenic curvature of the colon following an L3-L4 and L4-L4 XLIF for degenerative disc disease [43]. The patient experienced peritonitis and underwent an exploratory laparotomy that identified the colonic perforation, and a colostomy was maintained for 3 months after which the patient fully recovered. Tormenti et al. described a cecal perforation during the transpsoas approach of an XLIF for treating adult degenerative thoracolumbar scoliosis [44]. The patient underwent an emergency exploratory laparotomy and segmental bowel resection and recovered uneventfully.

Finally, delayed incisional hernias have been described following XLIF. Plato-Bello et al. reported the development of an abdominal pseudohernia requiring surgical repair 5 months after an uneventful L3-L4 LLIF [45]. Similarly, Gundanna and Shah presented a patient who exhibited herniation of abdominal contents through the original incision site 2 years after an L3-L4 XLIF and required laparoscopic hernia repair surgery [46].

7. Postoperative course and recovery

The postoperative course of XLIF surgery has been shown to minimize complications and recovery time. A prospective study of 600 patients treated with XLIF surgery revealed an average inpatient length of stay (LOS) of 1.21 days, and empirical evidence suggests that many patients may be able to ambulate within a day of the operation [47]. A similar study with a smaller cohort of 84 patients demonstrated a mean LOS of 2.6 days, with robust evidence of successful fusion on follow-up imaging [48].

On a comparable note, patient pain outcomes have been shown to significantly improve following the XLIF procedure. Improvements in two independent pain scoring metrics, the first being the visual analog scale (VAS) and the second being the Oswestry Disability Index (ODI), have been demonstrated in the literature. Specifically, a 2010 study by Youssef et al. reported a 77% and 56% increase in VAS and ODI respectively following XLIF at one-year follow-up [48]. Similarly, a 2011 study by Rodgers et al. demonstrated a 65% immediate improvement in VAS following XLIF, with 86.7% of patients satisfied with their operation at one-year follow-up [47]. The findings of both studies, with respect to improvements in patient-reported pain outcomes following XLIF, have been explored further and confirmed in several contemporary studies with similar conclusions [49, 50].

However, a major complication to consider following XLIF is graft subsidence, which threatens the long-term efficacy of the procedure. Several studies have demonstrated high rates of cage subsidence, as defined as >2 mm of cage settlement into the vertebral body, following the XLIF procedure [51, 52]. In many of these cases, 18-mm-wide and 22-mm-wide cages are used, and although previous studies have demonstrated their relative safety and efficacy, the rates of reported cage subsidence at these dimensions is suboptimal. A recent study by Lang et al. demonstrated that 26-mm-wide may reduce rates of cage subsidence while achieving excellent outcomes on both radiologic and clinical follow-up evaluation [53].

8. Advantages and disadvantages over similar techniques

The XLIF is a relatively new technique that is being quickly added into the toolkits of spine surgeons around the world. However, despite the rapid adoption of this surgical approach, there are both advantages and disadvantages to this technique compared to conventional approaches such as ALIF, TLIF, PLIF, and OLIF.

8.1 Advantages

One of the primary advantages to MIS surgery is the usage of smaller incisions compared to the large posterior or anterior approaches, resulting in reduced soft tissue damage, faster recovery times, and less postoperative pain. Multiple studies have described average hospital stays of just over 1 day and relatively few complications with XLIF [47, 49, 54, 55]. Additionally, unlike the ALIF, the XLIF is associated with less intraoperative blood loss [48] and lower risk of vascular injury, as major vessels such as the aorta are altogether avoided. For this reason, the XLIF conveniently eliminates the need for a vascular surgeon to either perform the ALIF approach or be on standby, which may translate to significant cost-savings. Furthermore, while there is increased risk of vascular damage in obese patient undergoing ALIF, this complication can be largely avoided by using the XLIF [56]. The XLIF also theoretically places the superior hypogastric plexus at risk, but there have been no cases of retrograde ejaculation compared to ALIF [57, 58]. Finally, the XLIF has been radiographically shown to have high rates of fusion, patient satisfaction, and patient-reported outcomes in several large studies [49, 54].

8.2 Disadvantages

Several reviews have noted that XLIFs are associated with a far higher rate of lumbar nerve root/plexus injury compared to alternatives [59], though other studies suggest that these rates are statistically comparable in XLIFs and ALIFs [60]. Furthermore, the XLIF approach requires dissection of the psoas muscle unlike in similar alternatives such as the OLIF or ALIF. The transpsoas approach leads to traumatic soft tissue damage, and coupled with the proximity of the genitofemoral nerve, likely explains the prevalence of transient thigh numbness/weakness. However, this complication has been largely shown to be temporary and clinically insignificant. Smaller studies have cited higher rates of prolonged hospital stay or complications [61], but these findings are out of the norm and may reflect surgeon inexperience or the learning curve associated with newer MIS techniques. Finally, studies have suggested that XLIFs are susceptible to intervertebral cage settling, which may lead to poorer long-term surgical correction and necessitate wider cages [62]. Even so, however, XLIFs are at significant risk of anterior and lateral protrusion, suggesting the need to reduced cage length whenever possible [63]. The XLIF is still a procedure in its early stages of implementation and higher quality evidence is needed to further differentiate it from alternative surgical approaches.

9. Patient perceptions

While more research is needed to further quantify the advantages and disadvantages of XLIF compared to conventional approaches, patient perceptions and expectations play an important role in the utilization of this newer technique. Presently, no study has investigated the role and impact of patient requests and perceptions in the decision-making process for which specific surgical approach is ultimately performed for lumbar spine pathologies. However, a recent study conducted by Narain et al. [64] found that prospective spine surgery patients with degenerative spine disorders overwhelmingly preferred a minimally invasive approach. These patients perceived open surgery to be more painful, having a higher complication rate, having prolonged recovery time, more expensive, and requiring heavier sedation compared to MIS. While this study clearly suggests that offering minimally invasive procedures is a highly marketable skill for spine surgeons, it also highlights the importance of setting realistic patient expectations for the operative and postoperative course. Spine surgeons will need to attenuate patient perceptions in the clinic with unbiased discussions on the advantages and disadvantages of XLIF compared to alternative approaches in the joint decision-making process to ensure proper clinical management.

10. Conclusion

The presence of minimally invasive spine surgery techniques in all practice settings has greatly increased over the past decade and will likely continue to rise in popularity due to patient requests/perceptions, marketability of MIS procedures, improving technology, and increased surgeon comfort. As MIS spine procedures become a standardized part of spine training, it will be important to continue monitoring the long-term advantages and disadvantages of procedures such as the XLIF compared to conventional approaches. Far more research is needed to determine the role of MIS techniques in a spine surgeon's armamentarium and whether specific surgery-related risks are justified by improved surgical and patient-reported outcomes. In the meantime, spine surgeons offering MIS procedures will need to provide transparent information regarding these surgeries to their patients, setting the expectation that these newer techniques may not necessarily result in superior outcomes compared to classic approaches.

Author details

Ronald Sahyouni, Luis D. Diaz-Aguilar and Donald Blaskiewicz*
Department of Neurosurgery, University of California, San Diego, United States

*Address all correspondence to: dblaskiewicz@health.ucsd.edu

IntechOpen

References

[1] Kalanithi PS, Patil CG, Boakye M. National complication rates and disposition after posterior lumbar fusion for acquired spondylolisthesis. Spine. 2009;34(18):1963-1969.

[2] DiPaola CP, Molinari RW. Posterior lumbar interbody fusion. *J Am Acad Orthop Surg*. 2008;16(3):130-139.

[3] Carreon LY, Puno RM, Dimar JR 2nd, Glassman SD, Johnson JR. Perioperative complications of posterior lumbar decompression and arthrodesis in older adults. *J Bone Joint Surg Am*. 2003;85(11):2089-2092.

[4] Scaduto AA, Gamradt SC, Yu WD, Huang J, Delamarter RB, Wang JC. Perioperative complications of threaded cylindrical lumbar interbody fusion devices: anterior versus posterior approach. *J Spinal Disord Tech*. 2003;16(6):502-507.

[5] Rihn JA, Patel R, Makda J, et al. Complications associated with single-level transforaminal lumbar interbody fusion. *Spine J*. 2009;9(8):623-629.

[6] Sasso RC, Best NM, Mummaneni PV, Reilly TM, Hussain SM. Analysis of operative complications in a series of 471 anterior lumbar interbody fusion procedures. Spine. 2005;30(6):670-674.

[7] Dhall SS, Wang MY, Mummaneni PV. Clinical and radiographic comparison of mini--open transforaminal lumbar interbody fusion with open transforaminal lumbar interbody fusion in 42 patients with long-term follow-up. *J Neurosurg Spine*. 2008;9(6):560-565.

[8] Park P, Foley KT. Minimally invasive transforaminal lumbar interbody fusion with reduction of spondylolisthesis: technique and outcomes after a minimum of 2 years' follow-up. *Neurosurg Focus*. 2008;25(2):E16.

[9] Kim CH, Easley K, Lee J-S, et al. Comparison of Minimally Invasive Versus Open Transforaminal Interbody Lumbar Fusion. *Global Spine J*. 2020;10(2 Suppl):143S -150S.

[10] Quante M, Halm H. [Extreme lateral interbody fusion. Indication, surgical technique, outcomes and specific complications]. *Orthopade*. 2015;44(2):138-145.

[11] Ozgur BM, Aryan HE, Pimenta L, Taylor WR. Extreme Lateral Interbody Fusion (XLIF): a novel surgical technique for anterior lumbar interbody fusion. *Spine J*. 2006;6(4):435-443.

[12] He Q. The Extreme Lateral Interbody Fusion (XLIF): Its Today and Tomorrow. *J Spine*. 2013;03(01). doi:10.4172/2165-7939.1000e112

[13] Pimenta L, Oliveira L, Schaffa T, Coutinho E, Marchi L. Lumbar total disc replacement from an extreme lateral approach: clinical experience with a minimum of 2 years' follow-up. *J Neurosurg Spine*. 2011;14(1):38-45.

[14] Mobbs RJ, Phan K, Malham G, Seex K, Rao PJ. Lumbar interbody fusion: techniques, indications and comparison of interbody fusion options including PLIF, TLIF, MI-TLIF, OLIF/ATP, LLIF and ALIF. *J Spine Surg*. 2015;1(1):2-18.

[15] Hah R, Kang HP. Lateral and Oblique Lumbar Interbody Fusion-Current Concepts and a Review of Recent Literature. *Curr Rev Musculoskelet Med*. Published online June 22, 2019:305-310.

[16] Tohmeh, A.G., W.B. Rodgers, and M.D. Peterson, *Dynamically evoked, discrete-threshold electromyography in the extreme lateral interbody fusion approach*. J Neurosurg Spine, 2011. **14**(1): p. 31-37.

[17] Uribe, J.S., et al., *Defining the safe working zones using the minimally invasive*

lateral retroperitoneal transpsoas approach: an anatomical study. J Neurosurg Spine, 2010. **13**(2): p. 260-266.

[18] Smith WD, Dakwar E, Le TV, Christian G, Serrano S, Uribe JS. Minimally invasive surgery for traumatic spinal pathologies: a mini-open, lateral approach in the thoracic and lumbar spine. Spine. 2010;35 (26 Suppl):S338-S346.

[19] Arnold PM, Anderson KK, McGuire RA Jr. The lateral transpsoas approach to the lumbar and thoracic spine: A review. *Surg Neurol Int*. 2012;3(Suppl 3):S198-S215.

[20] Hijji FY, Narain AS, Bohl DD, et al. Lateral lumbar interbody fusion: a systematic review of complication rates. *Spine J*. 2017;17(10):1412-1419.

[21] He L, Kang Z, Tang W-J, Rong L-M. A MRI study of lumbar plexus with respect to the lateral transpsoas approach to the lumbar spine. *Eur Spine J*. 2015;24(11):2538-2545.

[22] Anloague PA, Huijbregts P. Anatomical variations of the lumbar plexus: a descriptive anatomy study with proposed clinical implications. *J Man Manip Ther*. 2009;17(4):e107-e114.

[23] Banagan K, Gelb D, Poelstra K, Ludwig S. Anatomic mapping of lumbar nerve roots during a direct lateral transpsoas approach to the spine: a cadaveric study. Spine. 2011;36(11):E687-E691.

[24] O'Brien JR. Nerve Injury in Lateral Lumbar Interbody Fusion. *Spine*. 2017;42 Suppl 7:S24.

[25] Uribe JS, Isaacs RE, Youssef JA, et al. Can triggered electromyography monitoring throughout retraction predict postoperative symptomatic neuropraxia after XLIF? Results from a prospective multicenter trial. *Eur Spine J*. 2015;24 Suppl 3:378-385.

[26] Sedra F, Lee R, Dominguez I, Wilson L. Neurological complications using a novel retractor system for direct lateral minimally invasive lumbar interbody fusion. *J Clin Neurosci*. 2016;31:81-87.

[27] Nunley P, Sandhu F, Frank K, Stone M. Neurological Complications after Lateral Transpsoas Approach to Anterior Interbody Fusion with a Novel Flat-Blade Spine-Fixed Retractor. *Biomed Res Int*. 2016;2016:8450712.

[28] Abel NA, Januszewski J, Vivas AC, Uribe JS. Femoral nerve and lumbar plexus injury after minimally invasive lateral retroperitoneal transpsoas approach: electrodiagnostic prognostic indicators and a roadmap to recovery. *Neurosurg Rev*. 2018;41(2):457-464.

[29] Cahill KS, Martinez JL, Wang MY, Vanni S, Levi AD. Motor nerve injuries following the minimally invasive lateral transpsoas approach. *J Neurosurg Spine*. 2012;17(3):227-231.

[30] Benglis DM, Vanni S, Levi AD. An anatomical study of the lumbosacral plexus as related to the minimally invasive transpsoas approach to the lumbar spine. *J Neurosurg Spine*. 2009;10(2):139-144.

[31] Davis TT, Bae HW, Mok JM, Rasouli A, Delamarter RB. Lumbar plexus anatomy within the psoas muscle: implications for the transpsoas lateral approach to the L4-L5 disc. *J Bone Joint Surg Am*. 2011;93(16):1482-1487.

[32] Grimm BD, Leas DP, Poletti SC, Johnson DR 2nd. Postoperative Complications Within the First Year After Extreme Lateral Interbody Fusion: Experience of the First 108 Patients. *Clin Spine Surg*. 2016;29(3):E151-E156.

[33] Papanastassiou ID, Eleraky M, Vrionis FD. Contralateral femoral nerve compression: An unrecognized complication after extreme lateral

interbody fusion (XLIF). *J Clin Neurosci*. 2011;18(1):149-151.

[34] Peiró-García A, Domínguez-Esteban I, Alía-Benítez J. Retroperitoneal hematoma after using the extreme lateral interbody fusion (XLIF) approach: Presentation of a case and a review of the literature. *Rev Esp Cir Ortop Traumatol*. 2016;60(5):330-334.

[35] Santillan A, Patsalides A, Gobin YP. Endovascular embolization of iatrogenic lumbar artery pseudoaneurysm following extreme lateral interbody fusion (XLIF). *Vasc Endovascular Surg*. 2010;44(7):601-603.

[36] Assina R, Majmundar NJ, Herschman Y, Heary RF. First report of major vascular injury due to lateral transpsoas approach leading to fatality. *J Neurosurg Spine*. 2014;21(5):794-798.

[37] Fujibayashi S, Otsuki B, Kimura H, Tanida S, Masamoto K, Matsuda S. Preoperative assessment of the ureter with dual-phase contrast-enhanced computed tomography for lateral lumbar interbody fusion procedures. *J Orthop Sci*. 2017;22(3):420-424.

[38] Davis TT, Hynes RA, Fung DA, et al. Retroperitoneal oblique corridor to the L2-S1 intervertebral discs in the lateral position: an anatomic study. *J Neurosurg Spine*. 2014;21(5):785-793.

[39] Quillo-Olvera J, Lin G-X, Jo H-J, Kim J-S. Complications on minimally invasive oblique lumbar interbody fusion at L2-L5 levels: a review of the literature and surgical strategies. *Ann Transl Med*. 2018;6(6):101.

[40] Lee H-J, Kim J-S, Ryu K-S, Park CK. Ureter Injury as a Complication of Oblique Lumbar Interbody Fusion. *World Neurosurg*. 2017;102:693.e7-e693.e14.

[41] Kubota G, Orita S, Umimura T, Takahashi K, Ohtori S. Insidious intraoperative ureteral injury as a complication in oblique lumbar interbody fusion surgery: a case report. *BMC Res Notes*. 2017;10(1):193.

[42] Abe K, Orita S, Mannoji C, et al. Perioperative Complications in 155 Patients Who Underwent Oblique Lateral Interbody Fusion Surgery: Perspectives and Indications From a Retrospective, Multicenter Survey. *Spine*. 2017;42(1):55-62.

[43] Balsano M, Carlucci S, Ose M, Boriani L. A case report of a rare complication of bowel perforation in extreme lateral interbody fusion. *Eur Spine J*. 2015;24 Suppl 3:405-408.

[44] Tormenti MJ, Maserati MB, Bonfield CM, Okonkwo DO, Kanter AS. Complications and radiographic correction in adult scoliosis following combined transpsoas extreme lateral interbody fusion and posterior pedicle screw instrumentation. *Neurosurg Focus*. 2010;28(3):E7.

[45] Plata-Bello J, Roldan H, Brage L, Rahy A, Garcia-Marin V. Delayed Abdominal Pseudohernia in Young Patient After Lateral Lumbar Interbody Fusion Procedure: Case Report. *World Neurosurg*. 2016;91:671.e13-e16.

[46] Gundanna M, Shah K. Delayed Incisional Hernia Following Minimally Invasive Trans-Psoas Lumbar Spine Surgery: Report of a Rare Complication and Management. *Int J Spine Surg*. 2018;12(2):126-130.

[47] Rodgers WB, Gerber EJ, Patterson J. Intraoperative and early postoperative complications in extreme lateral interbody fusion: an analysis of 600 cases. Spine. 2011;36(1):26-32.

[48] Youssef JA, McAfee PC, Patty CA, et al. Minimally invasive surgery: lateral approach interbody fusion: results and review. Spine. 2010;35(26 Suppl):S302-S311.

[49] Phillips FM, Isaacs RE, Rodgers WB, et al. Adult degenerative scoliosis treated with XLIF: clinical and radiographical results of a prospective multicenter study with 24-month follow-up. Spine. 2013;38(21):1853-1861.

[50] Ahmadian A, Verma S, Mundis GM Jr, Oskouian RJ Jr, Smith DA, Uribe JS. Minimally invasive lateral retroperitoneal transpsoas interbody fusion for L4-5 spondylolisthesis: clinical outcomes. *J Neurosurg Spine*. 2013;19(3):314-320.

[51] Marchi L, Abdala N, Oliveira L, Amaral R, Coutinho E, Pimenta L. Radiographic and clinical evaluation of cage subsidence after stand-alone lateral interbody fusion. *J Neurosurg Spine*. 2013;19(1):110-118.

[52] Marchi L, Abdala N, Oliveira L, Amaral R, Coutinho E, Pimenta L. Stand-alone lateral interbody fusion for the treatment of low-grade degenerative spondylolisthesis. *ScientificWorldJournal*. 2012;2012:456346.

[53] Lang G, Navarro-Ramirez R, Gandevia L, et al. Elimination of Subsidence with 26-mm-Wide Cages in Extreme Lateral Interbody Fusion. *World Neurosurg*. 2017;104:644-652.

[54] Rodgers WB, Gerber EJ, Patterson JR. Fusion after minimally disruptive anterior lumbar interbody fusion: Analysis of extreme lateral interbody fusion by computed tomography. *SAS J*. 2010;4(2):63-66.

[55] Deluzio KJ, Lucio JC, Rodgers WB. Value and cost in less invasive spinal fusion surgery: lessons from a community hospital. *SAS J*. 2010;4(2):37-40.

[56] Rodgers WB, Cox CS, Gerber EJ. Early complications of extreme lateral interbody fusion in the obese. *J Spinal Disord Tech*. 2010;23(6):393-397.

[57] Sasso RC, Kenneth Burkus J, LeHuec J-C. Retrograde ejaculation after anterior lumbar interbody fusion: transperitoneal versus retroperitoneal exposure. Spine. 2003;28(10):1023-1026.

[58] Winder MJ, Gambhir S. Comparison of ALIF vs. XLIF for L4/5 interbody fusion: pros, cons, and literature review. *J Spine Surg*. 2016;2(1):2-8.

[59] Epstein NE. More nerve root injuries occur with minimally invasive lumbar surgery, especially extreme lateral interbody fusion: A review. *Surg Neurol Int*. 2016;7(Suppl 3):S83-S95.

[60] Hrabalek L, Adamus M, Gryga A, Wanek T, Tucek P. A comparison of complication rate between anterior and lateral approaches to the lumbar spine. *Biomed Pap Med Fac Univ Palacky Olomouc Czech Repub*. 2014;158(1):127-132.

[61] Knight RQ, Schwaegler P, Hanscom D, Roh J. Direct lateral lumbar interbody fusion for degenerative conditions: early complication profile. *J Spinal Disord Tech*. 2009;22(1):34-37.

[62] Tohmeh AG, Khorsand D, Watson B, Zielinski X. Radiographical and clinical evaluation of extreme lateral interbody fusion: effects of cage size and instrumentation type with a minimum of 1-year follow-up. Spine. 2014;39(26):E1582-E1591.

[63] Regev GJ, Haloman S, Chen L, et al. Incidence and prevention of intervertebral cage overhang with minimally invasive lateral approach fusions. Spine. 2010;35(14):1406-1411.

[64] Narain AS, Hijji FY, Duhancioglu G, et al. Patient Perceptions of Minimally Invasive Versus Open Spine Surgery. *Clin Spine Surg*. 2018;31(3):E184-E192.

Chapter 8

The Aspen MIS Spinous Process Fusion System

Tejas Karnati, Edwin Kulubya, Amir Goodarzi and Kee Kim

Abstract

The primary aim of this chapter will be to present an overview of the functionality and efficacy of the Aspen MIS spinous process fusion system, including a review of recent multicenter randomized data.

Keywords: Aspen, spinous process, posterior, lumbar, thoracic, spinal fusion, minimally invasive

1. Introduction

Over the last couple of decades, there has been a growing trend in the use of minimally invasive techniques in spine surgery because of low rates of complications, reduced hospital length of stay, lower estimated blood loss, and minimal soft tissue trauma [1]. With the growing prevalence of low back pain and lumbar degenerative spine disease, spine surgeons have found the need to expand their surgical armamentarium in treating degenerative spondylosis and spondylolisthesis [2]. Current surgical techniques to fuse two vertebral levels include posterolateral fusion, posterior lumbar interbody fusion (PLIF), transforaminal lumbar interbody fusion (TLIF), and extreme lateral interbody fusion associated with pedicle-screw fixation/instrumentation [3–7]; however, all these methods have drawbacks, such as increased operative time, risk of serious complications, and increased stiffness of the fused motion segment which may cause pathologic stresses at the adjacent levels [7]. These drawbacks of pedicle screw fixation (PSF) techniques have necessitated surgeons to explore novel and even more minimally invasive methods to achieve comparable levels of stability and fusion rates. Spinous process fixation (SPF)/interspinous process fixation (ISPF) achieved through the use of interspinous fusion devices (IFD) is not as widely used or known in the spine surgical community as PSF. Such devices aim to secure plates to the lateral aspects of two adjacent spinous processes thereby preventing motion at that segment. It is imperative that IFDs are not mistaken for similar other interspinous devices that offer "dynamic stabilization" such as X-STOP or DIAM etc. IFD placement has been successfully applied as an adjunct to posterolateral fusion and anterior fusion techniques and has shown similar rates of stability and fusion rates as PSF and has also been associated with improved or comparable patient-outcome scores [8].

In this chapter, we present the current evidence behind interspinous process fixation/fusion devices. We describe the primary biomechanical evidence and then present a discussion on clinical evidence of some case–control, case-series, and outcome studies. We then discuss the results of a recently completed randomized control trial of the Aspen® MIS Spinous Process Fusion System (Zimmer

Biomet Spine, Westminster, Colorado) and their implications in the use of IFDs in the future. At the end of the chapter, we describe in detail the components of the Aspen® MIS Spinous Process Fusion System and outline the basic surgical technique of placing this IFD successfully.

2. Evidence behind interspinous fusion/fixation devices

Ex-vivo biomechanical studies have demonstrated that IFDs provide comparable rigidity to PSF in flexion-extension [9]. The data are less clear in lateral bending and axial rotation. Techy et al. in 2013 specifically studied the Aspen interspinous device in comparison to pedicle screw fixation and found that the stability provided by the device was statistically equivalent to both bilateral or unilateral pedicle screw/ rod construct in flexion-extension; however, lateral bending and axial rotation tests showed pedicle screw fixation to have significantly greater stability [9]. In contrast, an earlier biomechanical study by Karahalios et al. in 2010 showed no difference in stability provided by IFDs compared to PSF in flexion-extension, lateral bending or axial rotation [10]. Papp et al. showed IFDs preserve adjacent facet joint anatomy [11]; other studies have even suggested IFDs may reduce load on intervertebral discs and potentially reduce the risk of adjacent segment disease [12, 13]. Yu et al. in 2014 studied their own novel IFD and found that interspinous process fixation combined with posterior lumbar interbody fusion (PLIF) was equivalent in biomechanical stability to bilateral pedicle screw/rod fixation with PLIF [14]. In short, it seems that cadaveric studies have shown IFDs to fare pretty well in restricting motion through flexion-extension comparable to the current gold-standard pedicle screw fixation but are likely unable to stabilize a motion segment against shearing forces.

Tomii et al. studied the S-plate (Kisco DIR, Osaka, Japan) in a series of 15 patients who underwent PLIF and subsequent IFD placement and found no complications and increase in mean JOA scores from 12.1 to 21.9 with a study follow-up period of 1.5–4 years [15]. Kim et al. showed decreased operative time for IFD placement and PLIF versus PS fixation and PLIF (135.8 minutes versus 170.8 minutes) and lower blood loss. The same study also showed decreased visual analog scale (VAS) scores in the immediate post-operative period of IFD and PLIF compared with PS and PLIF (4.6 vs. 7.0) [13]. However, VAS scores at 1 year follow-up showed no significant differences between the two groups. The Korean Oswestry Disability Index (ODI) scores also showed no significant differences between the two techniques [13].

To assess the value of IFDs in fusion rates, Vokshoor et al. [16] analyzed a sub-cohort of 50 patients who underwent IFD with PLIF or TLIF and showed 94% of them showed interspinous process fusion and 86% of those levels showed solid interbody fusion based on Burkus criteria [17]. Kim et al. [13] also studied fusion rates in their paper by either looking at 6-month post-operative flexion-extension films and/or assessing for trabecular bone on the 6 month post-operative CT scan; they found that IFD with PLIF showed a 92.5% fusion rate, which was similar to 91.6% fusion rates for PLIF with PS fixation. The same paper also reported adjacent segment disease in 12.5% of patients who underwent PLIF with IFD versus 36% in PLIF with PS fixation.

Lastly, Panchal et al. [8] in 2016 reported results from the first randomized, prospective, controlled, multi-center trial comparing outcomes from patients receiving anterior (ALIF) or lateral (LLIF) interbody fusion with adjunctive interspinous fusion with the Aspen® MIS device or pedicle screw fixation. Patients were followed pre-operatively and post-operatively at 6 weeks, 3 months, 6 months, 12 months, and even 24 months. The primary study endpoint was the comparison of the Oswestry Disability Index (ODI) score from the pre-operative time period to that of the 12-month post-operative time period. The primary hypothesis of the trial was noninferiority of the ODI score change by the Aspen® MIS IFD group (investigation) compared to the pedicle screw fixation group (control).

103 subjects underwent single-level interbody fusion via ALIF or LLIF approach. Sixty-six of them underwent adjunctive interspinous fusion with Aspen MIS spinous process fixation device. Thirty-seven of them were supplemented with pedicle screw fixation. All patients had degenerative disc disease and/or Grade 1 or 2 spondylolisthesis. The trial demonstrated no significant differences between the two groups with respect to patient-reported outcome scores (ODI, SF-36, or VAS) at 1.5, 3, 6, or 12-month time points. Interbody fusion was assessed at 12 months by evaluating computed tomography (CT) scans and scoring them according to the Brantigan, Stelfee, Fraser (BSF) criteria [18]; the authors found no significant difference in the BSF scores, even after adjusting for potential confounders such as anterolateral plating and/or interbody technique. Furthermore, 92% of the patients who had the Aspen® MIS device placed showed bone formation between the device plates bridging the spinous processes [8]. Operative times (47.6 minutes vs. 70.2 minutes), fluoroscopy times (12.2 seconds vs. 58.4 seconds), and blood loss (57.5 cc versus 103.7 cc) were also significantly less between the groups. Notably, no device breakage or dislodgement occurred in the study; however, 6 patients (3.1%) did have spinous process fractures and 3 patients (1.5%) needed to be reoperated due to new or worsening postoperative back and/or leg pain that may have been related to IFD placement.

In short, Panchal et al. was the first randomized multi-center trial to report that interspinous rigid fixation used as a supplement to anterior or lateral interbody fusion techniques is comparable to adjunctive pedicle screw fixation in terms of fusion rates and patient-reported outcomes and has a better intra-operative risk profile.

3. Aspen® MIS spinous process fusion system

The Aspen® Minimally Invasive Fusion System is a collection of spinous process fixation devices that are designed for rigid posterior fixation from T1 to S1 levels (see **Figure 1**). Each device consists of spinous process plates that come in three configurations (standard, medium, "Flared 5-1"), a "post plate" (a cylindrical device that is threaded in between the interspinous ligament and eventually joins

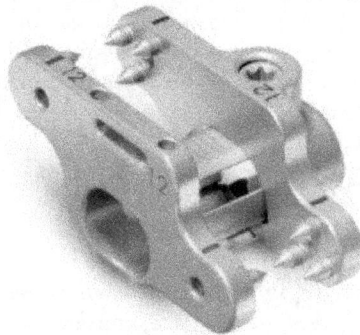

Figure 1.
Aspen® MIS fusion system standard size spinous process plate [19].

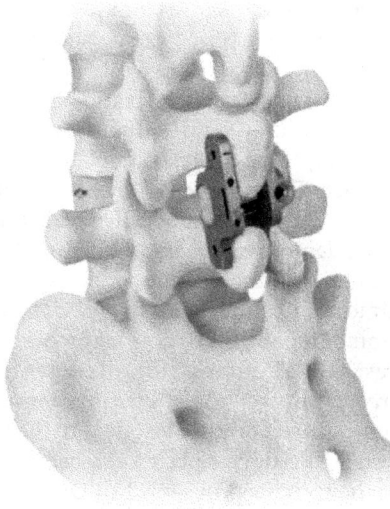

Figure 2.
Aspen® minimally invasive fusion system fully assembled [19].

the two spinous process plates) and a set screw that locks the system together. The cylindrical barrel in between the two plates can also hold approximately 0.5 cc to 3 cc of bone graft material. The system also has its own set of surgical tools to facilitate the insertion.

The final assembled Aspen® Minimally Invasive Fusion System interspinous fixation device is shown in **Figure 2**. The system is FDA approved and indicated for use in the United States as an adjunct to interbody and/or posterior fusion or as a standalone fixation device from T1 – S1 levels [8] in degenerative, traumatic, and deformity pathologies.

4. Surgical technique

The Aspen MIS system is placed with a patient in prone position through a 3–5 cm incision, enough to expose the length of the spinous process. Subperiosteal dissection is used to elevate the paraspinal muscles of the spinous process and lamina. The fusion site should be clear of connective and soft tissue then decorticated. The supraspinous ligament (SSL) can be removed or kept intact. Keeping the SSL intact helps preserves the natural anatomy and can prevent over distraction. The interspinous ligament is pierced as anterior as possible with a dilator (**Figure 3**).

A fluoroscopy image can be taken at this point to confirm anterior placement and appropriate level of dilator. The interspinous space is opened with a lamina spreader and measured to determine implant size. The interspinous space is decorticated with a rasp (**Figure 4**).

The barrel diameter is selected based on the fit of the rasp or spreader. The barrel length comes in a standard 21 mm size, appropriate for thick spinous processes or medium 18 mm when there are hypertrophied facets. The post plate implant is attached first to the left of the spinous process, then the barrel which is packed with graft material through the interspinous space, and finally the locking plate to the right of the spinous process (**Figure 5**).

Autograft and/or allograft can be placed posterior to the graft between the spinous process and across the lamina. The device should sit in the proper anterior

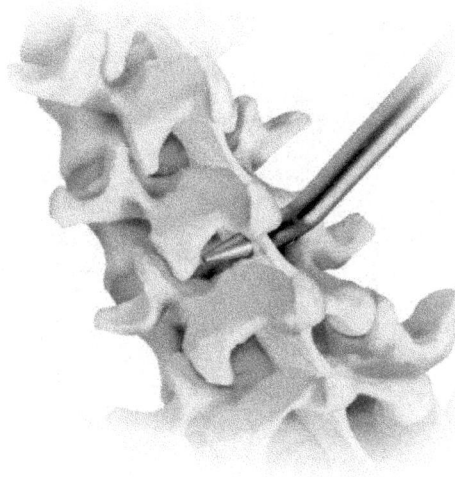

Figure 3.
Dilator is used to create space between the interspinous ligament [19].

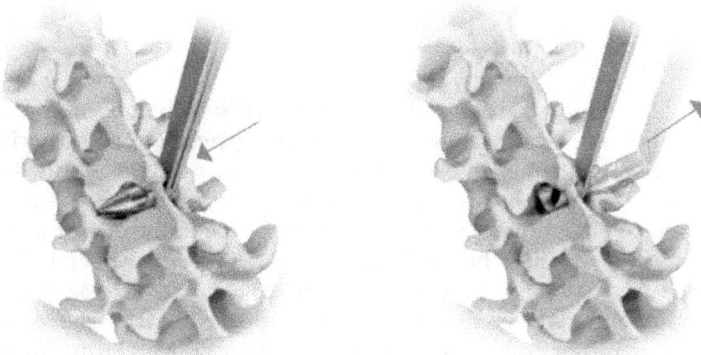

Figure 4.
Rasp for decortication [19].

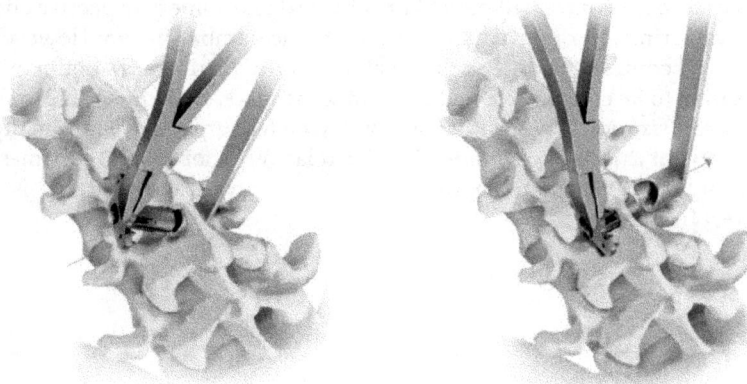

Figure 5.
Attachment of the post plate [18].

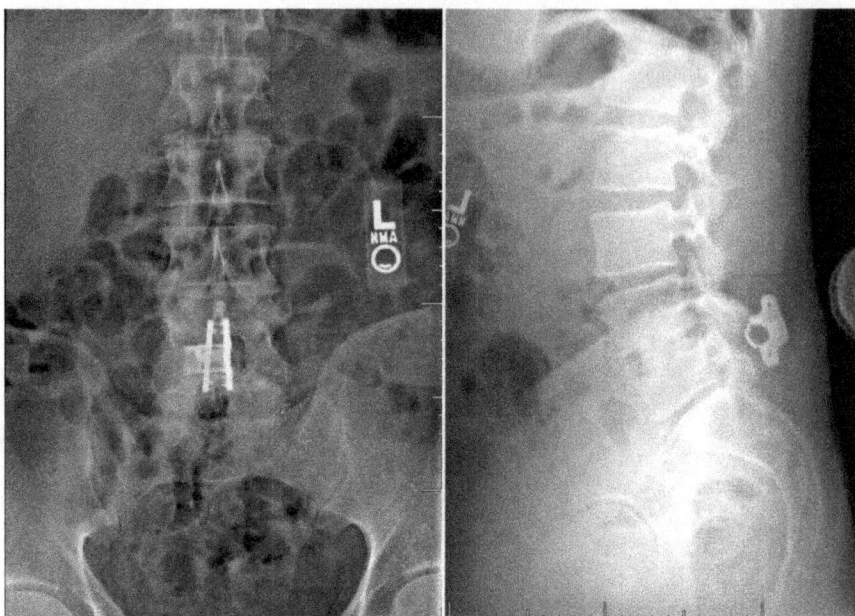

Figure 6.
A/P and lateral images of Aspen MIS fusion system at L4-L5.

placement and not protrude above the lumbodorsal fascia before compressing the plates and tightening the set screw. If the implant is placed too far posterior there is an increased risk of spinous process fracture. The spikes should be fully seated into the bone, but care should be taken to not over-compress and weaken the cortex.

The Aspen® MIS Fusion System should be removed in the case of nonunion or if any components loosen or break. The provided set-screwdriver or a T10 Torque driver can be used to loosen the locking set screw. The plates can then be lifted with a Cobb elevator and removed from the spinous process. **Figure 6** shows lateral and antero-posterior radiographs of a full assembled Aspen® MIS Fusion System.

5. Conclusion

Until recently, IFDs have had only biomechanical and some prospective clinic studies in evaluating their role as an adjunct to thoracolumbar fusion. However, the randomized control trial by Panchal et al. [8] showed outcomes of interspinous process fixation to be comparable and even, in some cases, more favorable to those of pedicle screw fixation. The relative ease with which a surgeon can minimally invasively implant this device combined with a relatively short operative times, low blood loss, and reduce hospital length of stay provides an attractive alternative to pedicle screw fixation.

Author details

Tejas Karnati, Edwin Kulubya, Amir Goodarzi and Kee Kim*
Department of Neurological Surgery, UC Davis School of Medicine, University of California, Davis, California, USA

*Address all correspondence to: kdkim@ucdavis.edu

IntechOpen

References

[1] Allen RT, Garfin SR. The economics of minimally invasive spine surgery: the value perspective. Spine. 2010;35:S375–S382.

[2] Freburger JK, Holmes GM, Agans RP, et al. The rising prevalence of chronic low back pain. Arch Intern Med. 2009;169(3):251.

[3] Weinstein JN, Lurie JD, Tosteson TD, et al. Surgical compared with nonoperative treatment for lumbar degenerative spondylolisthesis. Four-year results in the Spine Patient Outcomes Research Trial (SPORT) randomized and observational cohorts. J Bone Joint Surg Am. 2009;91:1295-1304.

[4] Resnick DK, Watters WC III, Mummaneni PV, et al. Guideline update for the performance of fusion procedures for degenerative disease of the lumbar spine. Part 10: lumbar fusion for stenosis without spondylolisthesis. J Neurosurg Spine. 2014;21:62-66.

[5] Karikari IO, Isaacs RE. Minimally invasive transforaminal lumbar interbody fusion: a review of techniques and outcomes. Spine. 2010;35:S294–S301.

[6] Raley DA, Mobbs RJ. Retrospective computed tomography scan analysis of percutaneously inserted pedicle screws for posterior transpedicular stabilization of the thoracic and lumbar spine: accuracy and complication rates. Spine (Phila Pa 1976). 2012;37(12):1092-1100.

[7] Amato V, Giannachi L, Irace C, Corona C. Accuracy of pedicle screw placement in the lumbosacral spine using conventional technique: computed tomography postoperative assessment in 102 consecutive patients. J Neurosurg Spine. 2010;12(3):306-313.

[8] Panchal R, Denhaese R, Hill C, et al. Anterior and lateral lumbar interbody fusion with supplemental interspinous process fixation: outcomes from a multicenter, prospective, randomized, controlled study. Int J Spine Surg. 2018;12(2):172-184.

[9] Techy F, Mageswaran P, Colbrunn RW, et al. Properties of an interspinous fixation device (ISD) in lumbar fusion constructs: a biomechanical study. Spine J. 2013;13:572-579.

[10] Karahalios DG, Kaibara T, Porter RW, et al. Biomechanics of a lumbar interspinous anchor with anterior lumbar interbody fusion: laboratory investigation. J Neurosurg Spine. 2010;12:372-380.

[11] Papp T, Porter RW, Aspden RM, et al. An in vitro study of the biomechanical effects of flexible stabilization on the lumbar spine. Spine. 1997;22:151-155

[12] Wang JC, Haid RW Jr, Miller JS, et al. Comparison of CD HORIZON SPIRE spinous process plate stabilization and pedicle screw fixation after anterior lumbar interbody fusion. Invited submission from the Joint Section Meeting On Disorders of the Spine and Peripheral Nerves, March 2005. J Neurosurg Spine. 2006;4:132-136.

[13] Kim HJ, Bak KH, Chun HJ, et al. Posterior interspinous fusion device for one-level fusion in degenerative lumbar spine disease: comparison with pedicle screw fixation - preliminary report of at least one year follow up. J Korean Neurosurg Soc. 2012;52:359-364.

[14] Yu X, Zhu L, Su Q. Lumbar spine stability after combined application of interspinous fastener and modified posterior lumbar interbody fusion: a biomechanical study. Arch Orthop Trauma Surg. 2014;134:623-629.

[15] Tomii M, Itoh Y, Numazawa S, et al. Spinous process plate (S-plate)

fixation after posterior interbody
fusion for lumbar canal stenosis due
to spondylolisthesis. Neurosurg Rev.
2013;36:139-143; discussion 43.

[16] Vokshoor A, Khurana S,
Wilson D, et al. Clinical and
radiographic outcomes after spinous
process fixation and posterior fusion
in an elderly cohort. Surg Technol Int.
2014;25:271-276.

[17] Burkus JK, Foley K, Haid RW,
et al. Surgical Interbody Research
Group—radiographic assessment of
interbody fusion devices: fusion criteria
for anterior lumbar interbody surgery.
Neurosurg Focus. 2001;10:E11.

[18] Fogel GR, Toohey JS, Neidre A,
Brantigan JW. Fusion assessment of
posterior lumbar interbody fusion using
radiolucent cages: x-ray films and helical
computed tomography scans compared
with surgical exploration of fusion.
Spine J. 2008;8(4):570-577.

[19] https://www.zimmerbiomet.com/
content/dam/zimmer-biomet/medical-
professionals/000-surgical-techniques/
spine/1079.2-US-en-REV1020_Aspen-
Surgical-Technique.pdf

Chapter 9

Application of Bone Morphogenetic Protein in Spinal Fusion Surgery

Siavash Beiranvand and Farshad Hasanzadeh-Kiabi

Abstract

Lumbar and cervical fusions are one of the most common types of spine surgeries performed globally with approximated 450,000 spinal fusion surgeries performed annually. (give reference) Bone Morphogenetic Proteins (BMPs) are secreted cytokines with several functions, within the TGF-b superfamily. BMP act as a disulfide-linked homo- or heterodimers and have been recognized as strong and effective regulators of important biological processes like formation and repair of osteocytes and chondrocytes, cell proliferation during embryonic development. Recombinant human bone morphogenetic protein 2 (rhBMP-2) is a very effective osteogenic growth factor that has been demonstrated to be effective in different types of spinal fusions and reduces the reliance on the use autologous iliac crest bone graft. In recent years there have been limitations regarding the use of rhBMP-2 because of issues like high costs, benefits, and safety issues about rhBMP-2. In this review, a comprehensive overview about the application of rhBMP-2 in spinal fusion surgery is given.

Keywords: Recombinant Bone Morphogenetic Proteins, Spinal fusion surgery, TGF-b, cytokines

1. Introduction

The use of osteobiologics to improve the outcome of spinal fusion has contributed to an increase in spinal fusion surgical procedures worldwide [1]. There are many different types of bone graft fusion materials currently on the market, however there is still a need for a cost effective biological material to achieve a successful permanent arthrodesis [2]. Presently iliac crest autograft, used for spinal fusion surgeries, is desirable as it possess osteo-biological properties with reduced risk of diseases transmission and graft rejection [3]. However, according to some studies, autograft has been linked to longer surgery time, few donor site availability [4], and chronic donor site pain [5, 6]. These limitations and disadvantages have led to novel therapeutic bone graft options for spinal fusion surgery [5, 7], like BMPs.

Marshall Urist was the first to describe BMP in 1965. It belongs to the transforming growth factor-ß family. There are various types of BMP molecules that exist, however few of them have been associated with osteoblast differentiation and bone development [7]. Recombinant rhBMP-2 is the market available form of

BMP-2 FDA approved for anterior lumbar interbody fusion (ALIF) [8]. There have been several clinical studies on the anterior lumbar interbody fusions and all have reported effective fusion rates, reduced operative time, reduced blood loss, and reduced hospital duration with the administration of rhBMP-2 when compared to iliac crest bone graft (ICBG) [9]. However, there have been conflicting reports as to whether rhBMP-2 is efficient in spinal fusion. A well-done study was performed by Papakostidis et al., who investigated the benefits of rhBMP-2 in promoting postero-lateral fusion. They concluded in their report that rhBMP-2 significantly increases rates of fusion, reduced hospital stay with the administration of BMP-2, compared to autologous iliac crest bone graft [10]. Lee et al. also confirmed the efficacy of the administration of rhBMP-2 in elderly patients undergoing posterolateral lumbar fusion at a single operative level [11]. Similarly, researchers like Meisel and colleagues also reported a 95–100% successful arthrodesis with use of BMP-2 when performing posterior lumbar interbody fusion [12]. However, recent systematic reviews question the efficacy and use of BMP-2 over iliac crest bone graft as noted in the Yale University Open Data base (YODA) Project and FDA reports. Including 13 randomized-controlled and 31 cohort studies, the study reported that for spinal fusion, rhBMP and iliac crest bone graft have similar efficacy. However, incidence of adverse event might be greater in anterior lumbar-body fusion and anterior cervical spine fusion. Furthermore, rhBMP can increase 24-month cancer risk [8]. These reports concluded that there were no substantial clear benefits of the administration of BMP-2 in spine fusion over autologous bone graft, and in fact there were more complications linked with BMP-2 use [13] (**Figure 1**).

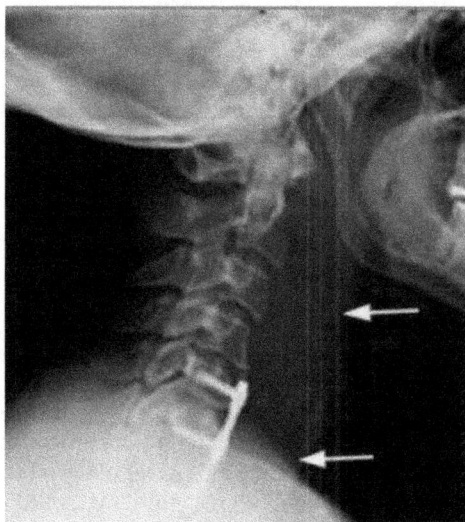

Figure 1.
Lateral radiograph of the cervical spine demonstrating massive soft- tissue swelling (arrows) following anterior cervical diskectomy and fusion surgery using rhBMP-2. Image was culled from.

2. Types of BMPs

There are about 20 different BMPs, however only BMP-2 is presently FDA approved for human spinal surgery [14, 15]. In addition, BMP-7 has been investigated for human use but is not FDA approved.

2.1 Different applications of rhBMP-2 in spinal fusion

2.1.1 Anterior lumbar interbody fusion

Burkus and colleagues demonstrated that patients administered with recombinant rhBMP-2 inside a Lumbar Tapered Fusion Device (LT-CAGE) had statistically significant lower length of surgery, lower duration of hospitalization and higher fusion rates at 6 months, 1 year and 2 years, compared to patients administered with the conventional ICBG [16]. In another clinical study, Burkus and co-worker compared the administration effect of rhBMP-2 in ALIF with structural cortical allografts and the INTER FIX Threaded Fusion Device to ICBG [17]. They concluded that patients administered with rhBMP- 2 exhibited better clinical and radiographic results, compared to ICBG patients [18]. Furthermore Burkus and colleagues reported that they recorded a superior and higher rates of radiographic fusion compared to the control group, in addition they demonstrated that rhBMP- 2 resulted into an improved ODI outcomes, enhanced radiographic fusion rate, compared to the ICBG control group. **Table 1** shows a summary of different available clinical studies demonstrating the potency of rhBMP-2 in increasing fusion rates of various spine surgeries.

2.2 Posterolateral lumbar fusion

The efficacies of rhBMP-2 have been studied and reported over the past few years. Boden et al. in their prospective randomized multicenter clinical trials demonstrated that the administration of rhBMP-2 in posterolateral lumbar fusion (PLF) [19]. They compared the effect of rhBMP-2 in patients with suffering from degenerative disc disease following PLF [20]. The patients were divided into three groups: autograft with pedical screw fixation, rhBMP-2 with pedical screw fixation, and rhBMP-2 without pedical screw fixation [21]. They concluded that they

Anatomical location of rhBMP-2	Adverse events	% Of fusion	Reference
Posterolateral lumbar	None reported	100%	[18]
Anterior lumbar	None reported	94.5%	[13]
Posterolateral lumbar	None reported	95%	[19]
Posterolateral lumbar	None reported	96%	[20]
Posterolateral lumbar	None reported	88%	[21]
Anterior lumbar	There were reports of retrograde ejaculation	NA	[22]
Posterior cervical	There were evidences of large seroma with recurrence after surgery	NA	[23]
Posterior lumbar interbody	Osteolysis	83%	[24]
Posterior lumbar interbody	There were reports of increased incidence of radiculitis	96.5%	[25]
Posterior lumbar interbody	There were reports malignancy at 5 years	NA	[26]

Culled from [27].

Table 1.
Showing the rates of fusion and adverse events associated with the application of rhBMP-2.

recorded a 100% fusion rate in the rhBMP-2 groups compared to the 40% fusion rate in the autograft group was 40.

Carreon and colleagues in their study, compared the application of autograft and higher dose rhBMP-2 in single-level of PLF case was carried out [22]. They concluded in their study that they recorded an 89% and 96% fusion rate in the autograft group and rhBMP- 2/CRM group respectively at 2 years follow-up. However they also recorded no similar clinical outcome measures between the two compared groups [23]. There have also been few smaller studies that reported related results of high fusion rates with the use of rhBMP-2 in PLF compared to ICBG [24].

2.3 Posterior lumbar interbody fusion

Haid and co-worker reported the efficiency of rhBMP-2 in posterior lumbar interbody fusion (PLIF), however there is a possibility for heterotopic bone formation. Haid and co-workers reported that they recorded 92.3% and 77.8% fusion rate with rhBMP-2 group and control group respectively, however there was an insignificant difference in clinical progress between the two compared groups [25]. They also reported via CT imaging that there was formation of ectopic bone around the PLIF [26].

2.4 Anterior cervical fusion

Baskin and colleague reported that there was a 100% fusion rate with the administration rhBMP-2 when compared with autograft [28]. Furthermore, they reported that the efficiency of rhBMP-2 was further improved when collagen sponges, PEEK cages, bioab- sorbable spacers, and allograft rings were added to it [29]. However, the positive results have been marred by reports of the incidence of soft-tissue related complications including potentially life-threatening airway compromise from tissue swelling. Cole, Veeravagu [30] conducted a MarketScan database-based retrospective study regarding the use of rhBMP in anterior cervical discectomy and fusion procedure. The outcomes of the study indicated that the use of drug is associated with increased incidence of hematoma, seroma, dysphagia, and pulmonary complications. Low dose rhBMP is also not associated with reduced incidence of the postoperative complications [31]. The FDA has placed a black box warning on the use of rhBMP-2 in the anterior cervical spine indicating that the risk of use may outweigh the benefit and therefore, its use is not recommended in anterior cervical fusion.

2.5 Transforaminal lumbar interbody fusion

There have been studies to investigate the efficiency of rhBMP-2 on transforaminal lumbar interbody fusion (TLIF, **Figure 2**). Villavicencio et al., in their clinical study on 74 patients, underwent single and multiple- level TLIF administered with rhBMP-2 and combined with auto- graft [33]. They recorded that there was radiographic evidence of fusion in all 74 patients after 10 months [34]. Furthermore, they recorded few adverse events in the rhBMP-2 group noting two patients developed postoperative radiculitis. In another similar study by Rihn et al., 48 patients underwent single-level TLIF administered with rhBMP-2 [35]. They concluded radiographic fusion, improved clinical outcomes and satisfaction with surgical results in 95.8%, 83% and 84% of the patients, respectively. However, 27.1% of their patients had complications like transient postoperative radiculitis and symptomatic ectopic bone formation (**Table 2**).

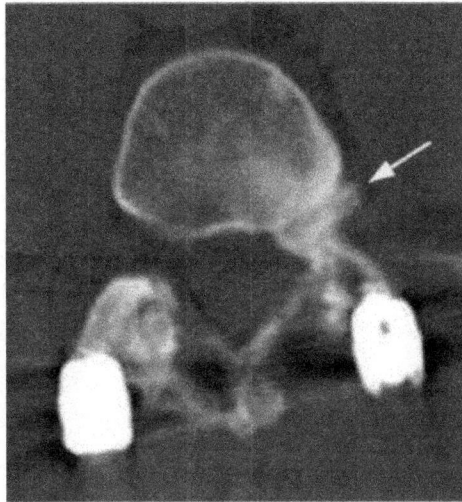

Figure 2.
An axial CT scan of the lumbar spine demonstrating ectopic bone formation (arrow) in the left neural foramen impinging on the exiting nerve root in a patient who underwent a transforaminal lumbar interbody fusion with rhBMP-2. Culled from [32].

Type of fusion	Recommendations
Anterior Lumbar Interbody Fusion (ALIF)	There have been reports of insignificant difference between the administration of rhBMP-2 and ICBG. It is recommended that in the absence of an autograft procedure, rhBMP-2 administration can be opted for.
Posterolateral Fusion (PLF)	There have been reports of no significant difference between the administration of rhBMP-2 and ICBG. It is recommended that in the absence of an autograft procedure, rhBMP-2 administration can be opted for.
Posterior Interbody Lumbar Fusion (PLIF)	The use of rhBMP-2 has been linked with formation of ectopic bone resulting into neurological deficit, as such ICBG procedure is preferred.
Transforaminal Interbody Fusion (TLIF)	The use of rhBMP-2 has been linked with seroma formation and neurological deficits. Judicious administration of rhBMP-2 is adviced

Culled from [36].

Table 2.
Showing alternative therapies to the use of rhBMP-2.

3. Conclusion

The use of rhBMP-2 offers an alternative therapeutic option when iliac crest autograft is either unavailable or may result in severe side effects. There are various clinical studies investigating how the use of rhBMP-2 can be effective in achieving spinal fusion. However, though rhBMP-2 is effective at achieving spinal fusion patients need to be informed of the possible formation ectopic bone requiring additional surgery and seroma formation when preforming transforaminal lumbar interbody fusion. There is a need for further study to minimize or lower the rates of complication linked with the application of rhBMP-2.

Conflict of interest

The authors deny any conflict of interest in any terms or by any means during the study.

Consent for publication

Informed consent was obtained from each participant.

Human and animal rights

No animals were used in this research. All human research procedures followed were in accordance with the ethical standards of the committee responsible for human experimentation (institutional and national), and with the Helsinki Declaration of 1975, as revised in 2013.

Availability of data and materials

All relevant data and materials are provided with in manuscript.

Contributors' statement page

Dr. Siavash Beiranvand: conceptualized and designed the study, drafted the initial manuscript, and reviewed and revised the manuscript. Designed the data collection instruments, collected data, carried out the initial analyses, and reviewed and revised the manuscript. **Dr.Farshad hasanzadeh-kiabi:** Coordinated and supervised data collection, and critically reviewed the manuscript for important intellectual content.

Author details

Siavash Beiranvand[1] and Farshad Hasanzadeh-Kiabi[2*]

1 Department of Anesthesiology, Faculty of Medicine, Lorestan University of Medical Sciences, Khorramabad, Iran

2 Department of Anesthesiology, Faculty of Medicine, Mazandaran University of Medical Sciences, Sari, Iran

*Address all correspondence to: dr.f.hassanzadehkiabi@gmail.com

IntechOpen

References

[1] Resnick, D.K., *Evidence-based spine surgery.* Spine, 2007. **32**(11): p. S15-S19.

[2] Carragee, E.J., E.L. Hurwitz, and B.K. Weiner, *A critical review of recombinant human bone morphogenetic protein-2 trials in spinal surgery: emerging safety concerns and lessons learned.* The spine journal, 2011. **11**(6): p. 471-491.

[3] Mroz, T.E., et al., *Complications related to osteobiologics use in spine surgery: a systematic review.* Spine, 2010. **35**(9S): p. S86-S104.

[4] Vahabi, S., et al., *Comparative study of 0.2% glyceryl trinitrate ointment for pain reduction after hemorrhoidectomy surgery.* The Surgery Journal, 2019. **5**(4): p. e192.

[5] Vahabi, S., et al., *Comparison of the Effect of Different Dosages of Celecoxib on Reducing Pain after Cystocele and Rectocele Repair Surgery.* The Open Anesthesia Journal, 2020. **14**(1).

[6] Vahabi, S., S. Beiranvand, and B. Radpay, The Incidence of Vasovagal Response in Spinal Anesthesia during Surgery.

[7] Cheng, H., et al., *Osteogenic activity of the fourteen types of human bone morphogenetic proteins (BMPs).* JBJS, 2003. **85**(8): p. 1544-1552.

[8] Fu, R., et al., *Effectiveness and harms of recombinant human bone morphogenetic protein-2 in spine fusion: a systematic review and meta-analysis.* Annals of internal medicine, 2013. **158**(12): p. 890-902.

[9] Burkus, J.K., H.S. Sandhu, and M.F. Gornet, *Influence of rhBMP-2 on the healing patterns associated with allograft interbody constructs in comparison with autograft.* Spine, 2006. **31**(7): p. 775-781.

[10] Papakostidis, C., et al., *Efficacy of autologous iliac crest bone graft and bone morphogenetic proteins for posterolateral fusion of lumbar spine: a meta-analysis of the results.* Spine, 2008. **33**(19): p. E680-E692.

[11] Lee, K.-B., et al., *The efficacy of rhBMP-2 versus autograft for posterolateral lumbar spine fusion in elderly patients.* European Spine Journal, 2010. **19**(6): p. 924-930.

[12] Meisel, H.J., et al., *Posterior lumbar interbody fusion using rhBMP-2.* European Spine Journal, 2008. **17**(12): p. 1735-1744.

[13] Simmonds, M.C., et al., *Safety and effectiveness of recombinant human bone morphogenetic protein-2 for spinal fusion: a meta-analysis of individual-participant data.* Annals of internal medicine, 2013. **158**(12): p. 877-889.

[14] Dawson, E., et al., *Recombinant human bone morphogenetic protein-2 on an absorbable collagen sponge with an osteoconductive bulking agent in posterolateral arthrodesis with instrumentation: a prospective randomized trial.* JBJS, 2009. **91**(7): p. 1604-1613.

[15] Moradkhani, M., et al., *Effects of Adjuvant Ketamine on Induction of Anesthesia for the Cesarean Section.* Current clinical pharmacology, 2020.

[16] Burkus, J.K., et al., *Anterior lumbar interbody fusion using rhBMP-2 with tapered interbody cages.* Clinical Spine Surgery, 2002. **15**(5): p. 337-349.

[17] Burkus, J.K., et al., *Use of rhBMP-2 in combination with structural cortical allografts: clinical and radiographic outcomes in anterior lumbar spinal surgery.* JBJS, 2005. **87**(6): p. 1205-1212.

[18] Boakye, M., et al., *Anterior cervical discectomy and fusion involving a*

polyetheretherketone spacer and bone morphogenetic protein. Journal of Neurosurgery: Spine, 2005. **2**(5): p. 521-525.

[19] Dimar, J.R., et al., *Clinical outcomes and fusion success at 2 years of single-level instrumented posterolateral fusions with recombinant human bone morphogenetic protein-2/compression resistant matrix versus iliac crest bone graft*. Spine, 2006. **31**(22): p. 2534-2539.

[20] Dimar, J.R., et al., *Clinical and radiographic analysis of an optimized rhBMP-2 formulation as an autograft replacement in posterolateral lumbar spine arthrodesis*. JBJS, 2009. **91**(6): p. 1377-1386.

[21] Boden, S.D., et al., *Use of recombinant human bone morphogenetic protein-2 to achieve posterolateral lumbar spine fusion in humans: a prospective, randomized clinical pilot trial 2002 volvo award in clinical studies*. Spine, 2002. **27**(23): p. 2662-2673.

[22] Carragee, E.J., et al., *Retrograde ejaculation after anterior lumbar interbody fusion using rhBMP-2: a cohort controlled study*. The Spine Journal, 2011. **11**(6): p. 511-516.

[23] Glassman, S.D., et al., *RhBMP-2 versus iliac crest bone graft for lumbar spine fusion: a randomized, controlled trial in patients over sixty years of age*. Spine, 2008. **33**(26): p. 2843-2849.

[24] Hamilton, D.K., et al., *Use of recombinant human bone morphogenetic protein-2 as an adjunct for instrumented posterior arthrodesis in the occipital cervical region: An analysis of safety, efficacy, and dosing*. Journal of Craniovertebral Junction and Spine, 2010. **1**(2): p. 107.

[25] Haid Jr, R.W., et al., *Posterior lumbar interbody fusion using recombinant human bone morphogenetic protein type 2* with cylindrical interbody cages. The Spine Journal, 2004. **4**(5): p. 527-538.

[26] Robin, B.N., et al., *Cytokine-mediated inflammatory reaction following posterior cervical decompression and fusion associated with recombinant human bone morphogenetic protein-2: a case study*. Spine, 2010. **35**(23): p. E1350-E1354.

[27] Even, J., M. Eskander, and J. Kang, *Bone morphogenetic protein in spine surgery: current and future uses*. JAAOS-Journal of the American Academy of Orthopaedic Surgeons, 2012. **20**(9): p. 547-552.

[28] Baskin, D.S., et al., *A prospective, randomized, controlled cervical fusion study using recombinant human bone morphogenetic protein-2 with the CORNERSTONE-SR™ allograft ring and the ATLANTIS™ anterior cervical plate*. Spine, 2003. **28**(12): p. 1219-1224.

[29] Helgeson, M.D., et al., *Adjacent vertebral body osteolysis with bone morphogenetic protein use in transforaminal lumbar interbody fusion*. The Spine Journal, 2011. **11**(6): p. 507-510.

[30] Cole, T., et al., *Usage of Recombinant Human Bone Morphogenetic Protein in Cervical Spine Procedures: Analysis of the MarketScan Longitudinal Database*. JBJS, 2014. **96**(17).

[31] Kukreja, S., et al., *Complications of Anterior Cervical Fusion using a Low-dose Recombinant Human Bone Morphogenetic Protein-2*. Korean Journal of Spine, 2015. **12**(2): p. 68-74.

[32] Rihn, J.A., et al., *The use of bone morphogenetic protein in lumbar spine surgery*. JBJS, 2008. **90**(9): p. 2014-2025.

[33] Humphreys, S.C., et al., *Comparison of posterior and transforaminal approaches to lumbar interbody fusion*. Spine, 2001. **26**(5): p. 567-571.

[34] Villavicencio, A.T., et al., *Safety of transforaminal lumbar interbody fusion and intervertebral recombinant human bone morphogenetic protein—2.* Journal of Neurosurgery: Spine, 2005. **3**(6): p. 436-443.

[35] Rihn, J.A., et al., *The use of RhBMP-2 in single-level transforaminal lumbar interbody fusion: a clinical and radiographic analysis.* European Spine Journal, 2009. **18**(11): p. 1629.

[36] Hustedt, J.W. and D.J. Blizzard, *The controversy surrounding bone morphogenetic proteins in the spine: a review of current research.* The Yale journal of biology and medicine, 2014. **87**(4): p. 549.

Chapter 10

Minimally Invasive Transforaminal Lumbar Interbody Fusion: A Novel Technique and Technology with Case Series

Mick Perez-Cruet, Ramiro Pérez de la Torre and Siddharth Ramanathan

Abstract

Minimally invasive spine surgery (MIS) transforaminal lumbar interbody fusion (MI-TLIF) has been utilized to treat a variety of spinal disorders. Like other minimally invasive spine surgery techniques and technology, the MI-TLIF approach has the potential to limit the morbidity associated with larger exposures required for open surgery. The MI-TLIF approach has a number of advantages over many other minimally invasive spine surgery approaches including direct decompression of neural elements, collection of morselized autograph from the surgical site to achieve high fusion rates, restoration of spinal canal diameter, foraminal diameter, disk height, and reduction of spondylolisthesis. In this chapter, we discuss a novel technique for performing MI-TLIF developed by the senior author who is a leading minimally invasive spine surgeon. The technique and technology illustrated in this chapter were developed out of a recognition of a need to reduce the learning curve for performing MI-TLIF, as well as need for a cost-effective method that provides a high fusion rate, excellent clinical outcomes, and low complication rate. The indications, surgical planning, postoperative care, complications, and patient outcomes in a large series will be reviewed using this novel MI-TLIF technique.

Keywords: minimally invasive spine surgery (MIS), minimally invasive transforaminal lumbar interbody fusion (MI-TLIF), degenerative disk disease, spondylolisthesis, lumbar stenosis, recurrent disk herniation

1. Introduction

Over the last two decade, the use of spine instrumentation options has become the standard of care for the treatment of a variety of spinal disorders [1–6]. Lumbar spine surgery indications continue to evolve as more clinical outcomes studies become available [7–10]. Indications include lumbar stenosis, lumbar spondylolisthesis with and without stenosis, degenerative disk disease (DDD), lumbar scoliosis, and recurrent disk herniations. There are a variety of surgical options including open fusion and instrumentation, posterior lumbar interbody fusion (PLIF), minimally invasive transforaminal lumbar interbody fusion (MI-TLIF), oblique lateral interbody fusion (OLIF), abdominal lumbar interbody fusion (ALIF),

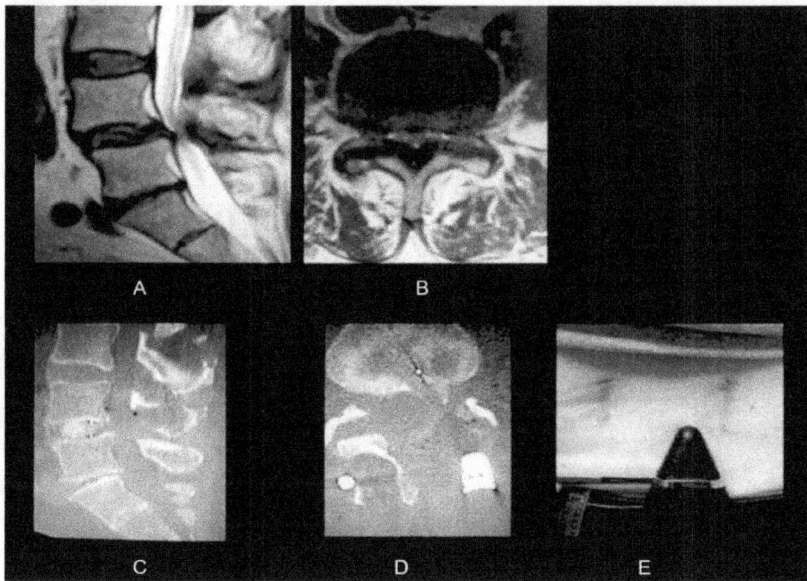

Figure 1.
Preoperative A. sagittal and B. axial T2-weighted MRI images showing L4–5 grade 1 spondylolisthesis with associated stenosis. Postoperative C. sagittal, D. axial CT, and E. postoperative incision following MI-TLIF approach showing adequate central canal decompression, restoration of disk height, and normal sagittal alignment.

extreme lateral interbody fusion (XLIF), and others. In this chapter, we will review a novel MI-TLIF technique, discuss surgical nuances related to the procedure, and review a large clinical series using this technique and technology.

MI-TLIF is a minimally invasive spine technique that has gained tremendous acceptance in the surgical community. The number of publications utilizing the MI-TLIF technique testifies to its popularity compared with other minimally invasive spine surgery (MIS) fusion techniques [11–13]. The rationale behind the MI-TLIF procedure is the advantage of direct neural decompression, reduced neural retraction during the procedure, and compression of interbody graft material to promote arthrodesis [14–16]. Additionally, the posterior approach permits collection of drilled morselized autograph bone for fusion material, which when placed into the intervertebral disk space promotes arthrodesis (**Figure 1**). Further, the technique and instrumentation that have been developed preserve the disk annulus and contain the injected bone graft material. By placing this bone graft material under load, arthrodesis is promoted according to Wolff's law. On comparative studies, MI-TLIF was shown to be superior to other techniques in terms of bone fusion rates, complications rates, and biomechanical properties [17–23]. Most of the proponents of this approach support the concept of preserved anatomical structures avoiding instability, while restoring sagittal alignment [24]. Using the same posterior approach, percutaneous pedicle screws can be applied bilaterally which further promotes fusion rates.

2. Indications for MI-TLIF

Indications for fusion and instrumentation include degenerative disk disease (DDD), spondylolisthesis with or without stenosis, lumbar stenosis, scoliosis, and instability due to trauma/tumor resection (**Figure 2**) [25].

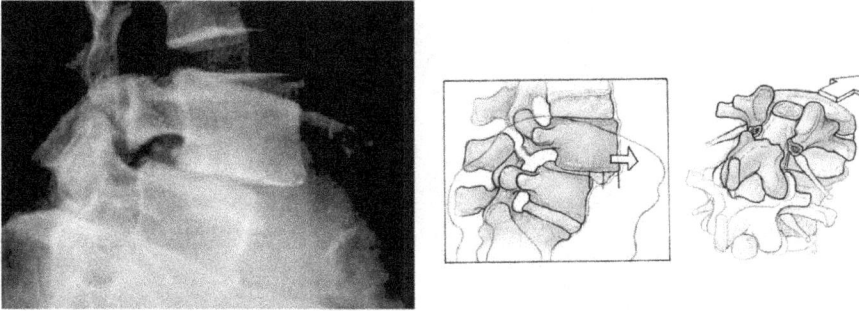

Figure 2.
Lateral plain X-ray radiograph and illustration of spondylolysis with pars interarticularis defect.

There a number of relative contraindications for selecting this approach including severe osteoporosis, active infection, and uncontrolled bleeding disorders. However, we have found that patients with osteoporosis can be effectively treated using this technique. Obesity was initially a relative contraindication; however, as more clinical outcomes studies, including our series, have become available, this can now be considered as an accepted indication when other techniques are not appropriate [26].

3. Surgical procedure

3.1 Preoperative planning

A thorough preoperative patient history and examination is performed. Preoperative radiographic workup includes plain X-rays with AP, lateral, flexion, and extension views. Magnetic resonance imaging (MRI) of the lumbar spine is performed. In reoperation cases or in patients with scoliosis, a computed tomography (CT) myelogram can be helpful in defining bony anatomy, foraminal, and central canal stenosis better. In patients without significant neural compression and relatively preserved disk height, lumbar diskography with post-diskography CT confirming annular tears can be a method to identify the origin of discogenic back pain that can respond favorably to interbody fusion [27].

3.2 Patient positioning

We prefer general anesthesia with endotracheal intubation for most patients as these cases average 3 hours. Once the patient is intubated, a Foley catheter is placed and the patient is log-rolled onto a Jackson table in the prone position (**Figure 3**). The Jackson table is helpful, because it allows unencumbered fluoroscopic visualization of the spine along with easy removal of the fluoroscopic unit from the surgical field. All pressure points are adequately padded. A time-out is called to confirm surgical level and procedure, proper padding of patient, etc.

3.3 Spinal approach

3.3.1 Incision

The patient is prone-positioned with appropriate padding, prepping, and draping in sterile surgical fashion. The midline is marked to help orient the surgeon. An

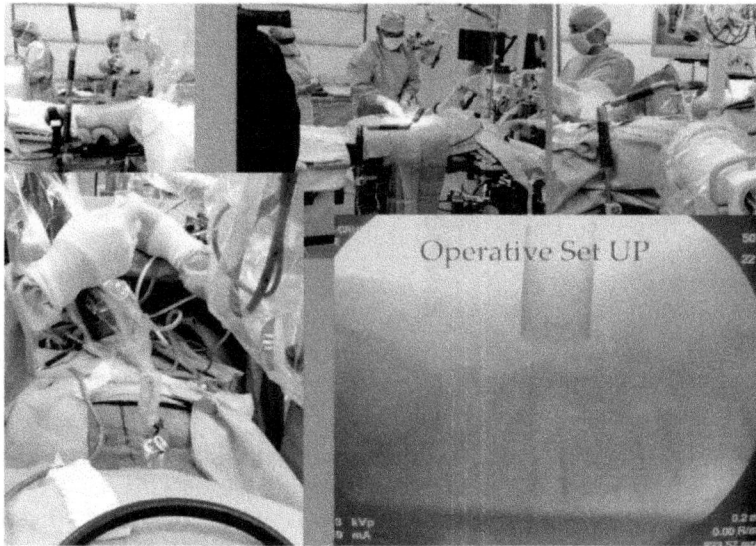

Figure 3.
Intraoperative images showing patient positioned prone on a Jackson table, fluoroscopic unit in place, and pneumatic arm used to holds the tubular retractor for easy repositioning at the press of a button.

18-gauge spinal needle is used with lateral fluoroscopy to identify the proper level. A 3–3.5 cm incision is made lateral to the midline directly over the disk space in which the MI-TLIF is to be performed. This distance from the midline allows access to the base of the spinous process for adequate minimally invasive laminectomy for direct decompression of the spinal canal. If no decompression is required, the incision is made 3.5 cm distance from the midline. This distance facilitates interbody implant placement within the disk space. After the fascial incision is made parallel to the spinous processes, the one-step-dilator is brought into the operating field (**Figure 4**). With the support of a holder and using fluoroscopic guidance, the dilator is advanced toward the facet in a clockwise fashion. After docking the dilator on the facet, counterclockwise rotation of the handle opens the flanges of the dilator, separating the muscle tissue. A tubular retractor of the appropriate depth is then placed. The procedure is performed under direct microscope visualization through the tubular retractor. The approach is bloodless and obviates the need for K-wires or serial dilation, avoiding the potential complications that can be seen when using these instruments (**Figure 4**).

3.3.2 Lumbar exposure and decompression

After positioning the tubular retractor, the microscope is brought into the surgical field. AP and lateral fluoroscopy can be used to ensure proper retractor placement. Soft tissue is excised to the extent of the facet laterally and the ipsilateral lamina medially, and a high-speed drill and M8 cutting burr are used to drill the lamina. All drilled bone is collected using the BoneBac™ Press (Thompson MIS, Salem, NH). This bone is used for fusion material, avoids graft site morbidity, and if needed, can be combined with other biologic material (**Figure 5**). If significant spinal stenosis coexists, a minimally invasive laminectomy is performed allowing circumferential decompression of the spinal canal. We are strong believers that decompression needs to be addressed before percutaneous screws are placed, as most of the surgical steps are done in a logical stepwise fashion.

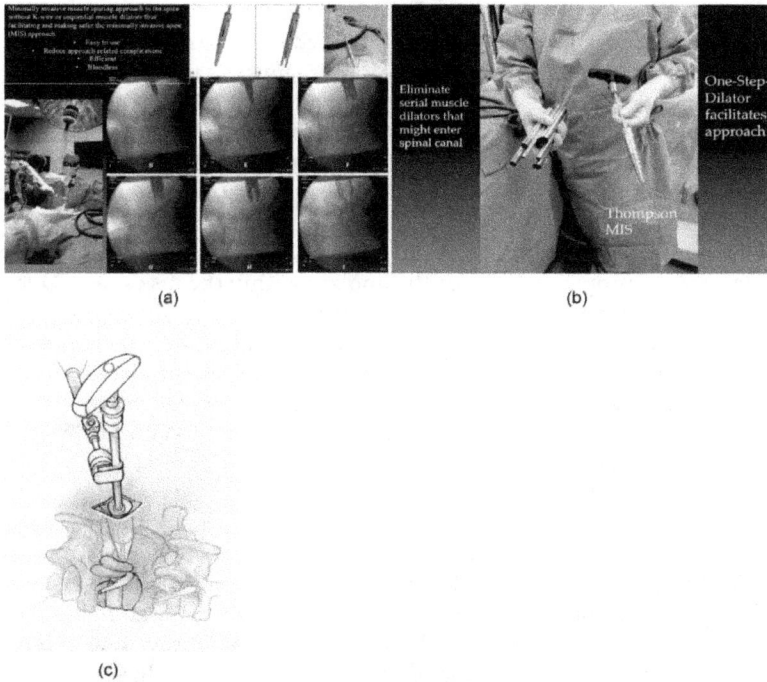

Figure 4.
a. Intraoperative images showing the use of one-step-dilator to approach the spine and b. eliminate K-wire and multiple muscle dilators. c. Illustration of the one-step-dilator retractor used to approach the spine in a muscle sparing fashion.

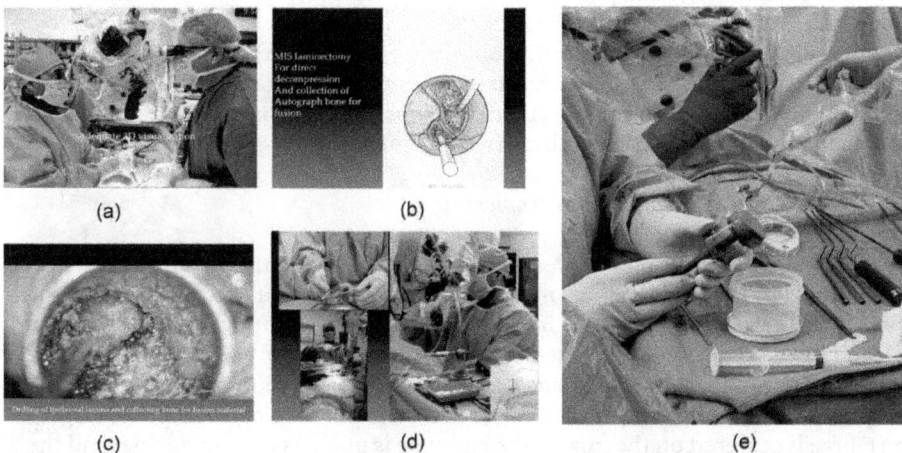

Figure 5.
a. Intraoperative view showing the use of microscope. b. Illustration, and c. intraoperative photos showing decompression of lamina with high-speed cutting burr and d. collection of drilled morselized bone graft material e. using the BoneBac™ press.

3.3.3 Interbody fusion

Upon decompressing the spinal canal, the tubular retractor is repositioned to expose the facet complex. In every case, lateral fluoroscopy is used to confirm the appropriate level. An ipsilateral facetectomy is then completed using a high-speed cutting burr, and an annulotomy is performed to enter the disk space. A series of disk space reamers, curettes, and rongeurs are used to prepare the disk space and vertebral endplates for interbody arthrodesis. Care must be taken to adequately remove the cartilage endplates to improve interbody arthrodesis. Once preparation of the disk space is completed, the implant is selected based on trials. The most commonly used implant size is 7 mm wide by 11 mm or 12 mm tall and 26 mm in length. This size appears to be appropriate in the majority of cases and provides for adequate disk and foraminal height restoration. In many cases, partial reduction of spondylolisthesis occurs with restoration of the disk height. Lateral fluoroscopic images identify the proper location of the implant within the disk space. Once the implant is within the disk space, the tubular retractor is positioned medially to help seat the implant within the center of the disk space. The relatively small width of the implant design and bulleted nose allows for ease of placement within the interbody disk space. The implant is then rotated 90 degrees thus restoring disk space and foraminal height to 11 or 12 mm, respectively. With the implant properly positioned, BoneBac™ TLIF bullets are filled with morselized autograph bone collected during the procedure using the BoneBac™ Press. The bone is then pushed down the handle of the implant to allow filling of the disk space as the bone is pushed out around the implant and contained by the intact annulus fibrosis of the disk. Typically, 10–12 bullets of drilled morselized autograph are used to completely fill the disk space. This process allows for off-loading of the interbody implant while allowing the compression of the morselized autograph to improve fusion rates via Wolff's law. If more bone graft material is needed, the morselized autograph is mixed with additional bone graft material (i.e. allograft, demineralized bone matrix, etc.). Once the disk space is packed with bone graft, the implant is released and deployed into the disk space. The disk space is inspected with a ball-ended probe under microscope visualization to assure that all bone graft material is within the disk space and that adequate direct neural decompression has been achieved. Additionally, bone graft material can be used to reconstruct the resected facet complex allowing for circumferential bone fusion (**Figure 6**). With complete and adequate hemostasis, the tubular retractor is removed allowing the paraspinous muscles to return to their normal anatomical position. Postoperative CT confirms adequate filling of disk space with morselized autograph.

3.3.4 Percutaneous pedicle screw instrumentation

Upon completion of decompression and interbody fusion, the tubular retractor is removed, and the paraspinous muscles are allowed to return to their normal anatomical position. A contralateral incision is made equidistant from the midline, and AP and lateral fluoroscopy are used to target the pedicles for percutaneous pedicle screw fixation. Alternatively, image-guided robotic navigation can be used for this purpose [28, 29]. To avoid parallax distortion on fluoroscopic imaging, the target vertebrae is centered on the image, the endplate is made as one single line, and the spinous process is oriented between the pedicles. Intraoperative electrophysiologic monitoring with EMG is performed (**Figure 6**). To ensure proper positioning after K-wire and pedicle screw placement, these constructs are stimulated with a probe. Stimulation thresholds less than 8 mAmps necessitate repositioning of K-wire and/ or pedicle screw. Typically, percutaneous screws are placed bilaterally and segmentally at each MI-TLIF section to ensure adequate fixation and promote arthrodesis. To reduce radiation exposure, we use the MinRad™ arm (Thompson MIS, Salem, NH) to hold the Jamshidi needle in place. This device also facilitates percutaneous pedicle screw placement by allowing for small adjustments of the pedicle targeting needle, thereby improving pedicle screw placement accuracy (**Figure 7**).

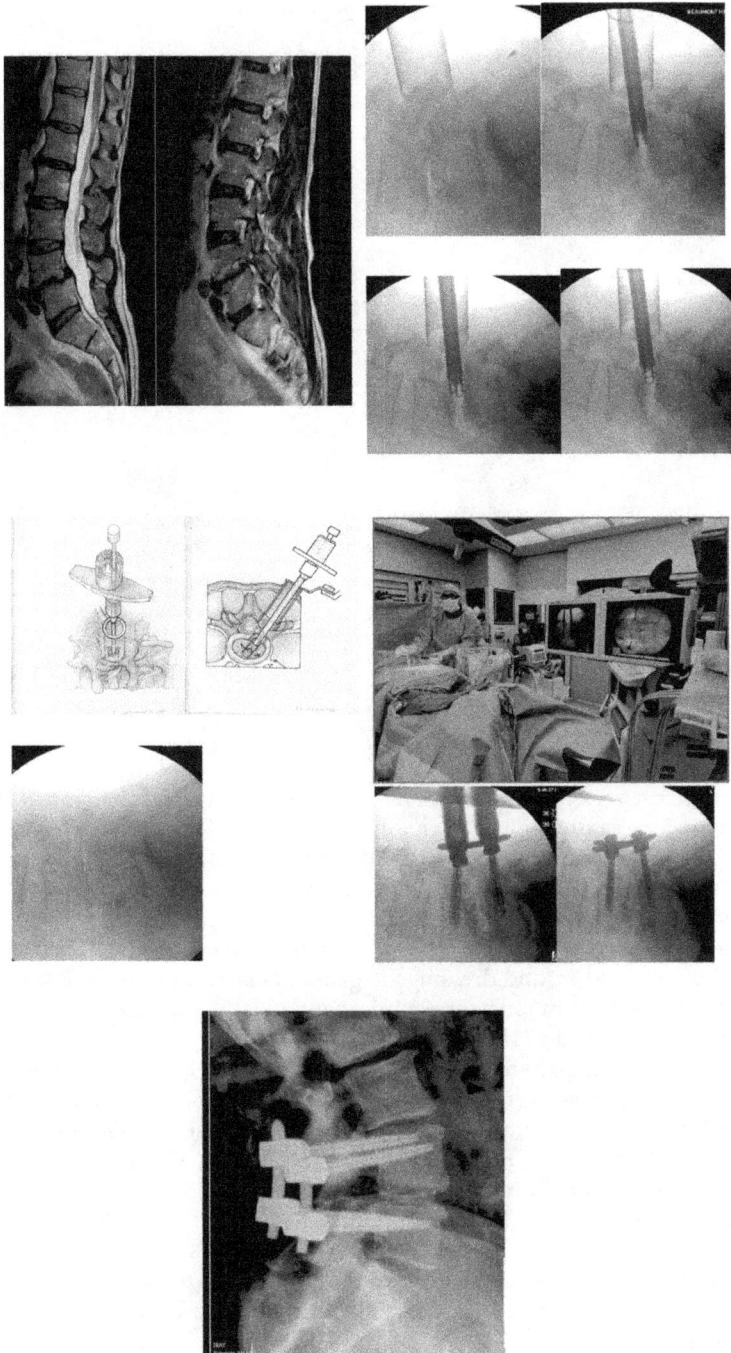

Figure 6.
Preoperative MRI showing A. midline and B. lateral sagittal images of grade 1 spondylolisthesis with severe foraminal stenosis causing patient's symptoms of debilitating back pain. Intraoperative fluoroscopic images showing C. tubular retractor in place, D. placement of 7 wide PEEK implant into the interbody space, E–F. rotation of the implant to restore disk height to 11 mm, G–H. injection of drilled morselized autograph into the disk space, I. deploying implant into the disk space, J. photo showing intraopertive stimulation of K-wires and percutaneous pedicle screws to assure adequate placement, K–L. reduction of the spondylolisthesis using percutaneous pedicle screw reduction methods, and M. final lateral fluoroscopic image using Thompson MIS BoneBac™ TLIF system. Note restoration of disk height, sagittal alignment, and foraminal and canal diameter.

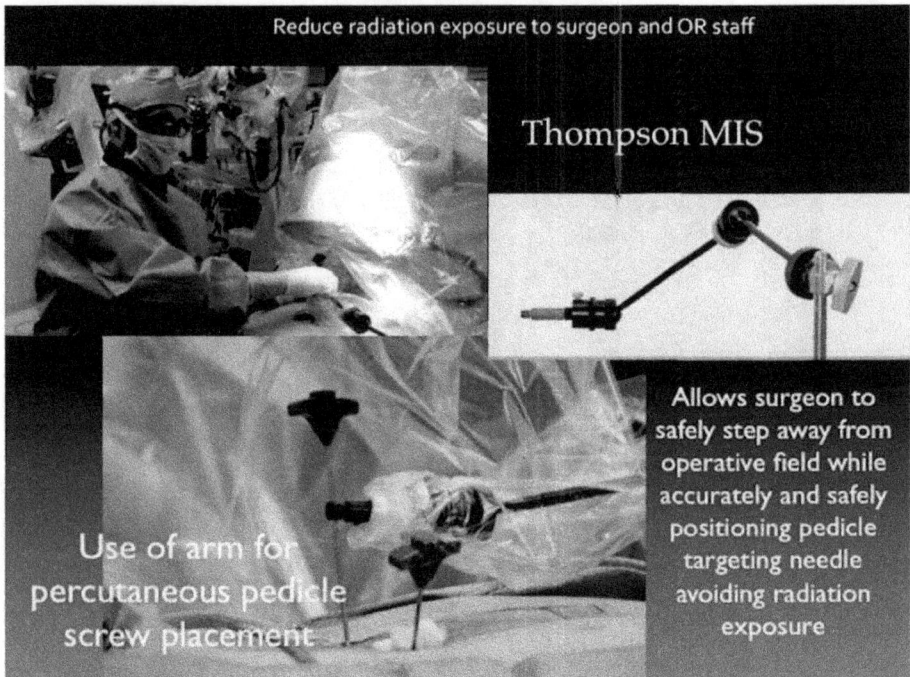

Figure 7.
Intraoperative photo and images of MinRad used to hold pedicle access needle for.

If concomitant vertebral subluxation is present, reduction of the spondylolisthesis is attempted to restore sagittal alignment (**Figure 6**). This technique significantly increases the neural foraminal size and central canal diameter while also ensuring sufficient surface area between adjacent vertebrae for arthrodesis (**Figure 8**).

After wound irrigation, a 2–0 vicryl suture is used to close the fascial layer in an interrupted fashion. A subcuticular stitch and skin glue adhesive are used to close the skin. Drainage and wound dressing are generally not required, and the infection rate is negligible. Excellent long-term clinical outcomes using this MI-TLIF technique have been achieved (**Table 1**) [26].

Excellent long-term patient-generated outcome results have been achieved using the MI-TLIF technique described. Source: Quality-of-Life Outcomes With Minimally Invasive Transforaminal Lumbar Interbody Fusion Based on Long-Term Analysis of 304 Consecutive Patients. Mick J. Perez-Cruet, MD, MS, Namath S. Hussain, MD, G. Zachary White, BS, Evan M. Begun, BS, Robert A. Collins, DO, Daniel K. Fahim, MD, Girish K. Hiremath, MD, Fadumo M. Adbi, BS, and Sammy A. Yacob, SPINE Volume 39, Number 3, p E191 - E198, 2014.

Adjacent segment disease over a 5-year postoperative period has been approximately 2% compared to 13.6% in traditional open lumbar arthrodesis series [8, 30].

3.3.5 Postoperative care

Patients typically stay in the hospital for 2–3 days after surgery and ambulate the day after surgery. Postoperative pain is managed initially with IV and oral pain medications and muscle relaxers as needed. Consultation with physical therapist or occupational therapist is arranged before discharge. Patients are discharged with postoperative care guidelines and follow-up plans. The follow-up is performed at

(a)

(b)

(c)

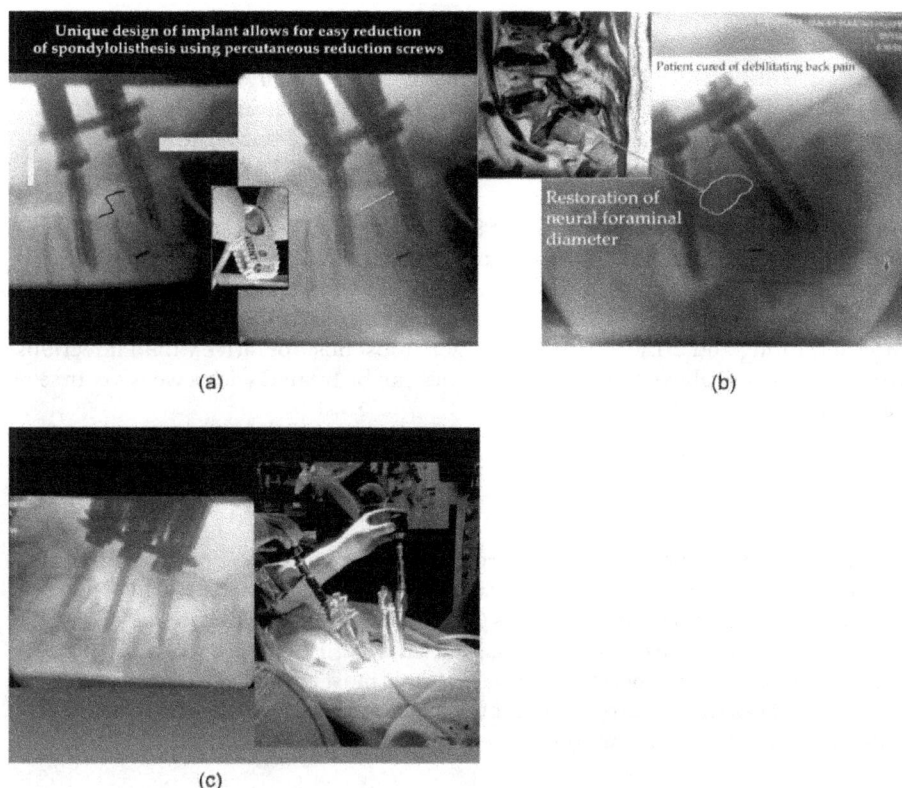

Figure 8.
a. Intraoperative lateral fluoroscopic images using unique design of the BoneBacTM TLIF device to reduce grade 1 spondylolisthesis to grade 0 and thus b. restore foraminal height allowing adequate decompression of the exiting nerve root. c. Reduction of multi-segmental spondylolisthesis with percutaneous reduction screws.

	Baseline	Follow-up time		
		12 mo*	24 mo*	47 mo*
Back pain visual analog scale	7.0 ± 2.4	4.2 ± 3.0 (2.8, 40%)	4.5 ± 3.0 (2.5, 35.7%)	3.5 ± 2.8 (3.5, 50%)
Oswestry Disability Index	43.1 ± 15.7	29.7 ± 18.8 (13.4, 31.1%)	30.2 ± 20.4 (12.9, 29.9%)	28.2 ± 21.7 (14.9, 34.6%)
SF-36 physical component score	30.6 ± 7.8	38.3 ± 11.3 (7.7, 25.2%)	38.1 ± 11.7 (7.5, 24.5%)	39.6 ± 11.7 (9, 29.4%)
SF-36 mental component score	43.8 ± 11.0	48.3 ± 13.0 (4.5, 10.3)	49.7 ± 12.9 (5.9, 13.5%)	49.7 ± 11.2 (5.9, 13.5%)
P		<0.001	<0.001	<0.05

The values are given as the mean and the standard deviation.
*SF-36 indicates Short-Form 36.*Net change and percent improvement from baseline, respectively, are in parenthesis.*

Table 1.
Long-term results.

2 weeks, 3 month, 6 month, and 1 year from the day of surgery. Patients are advised to wear a LSO brace when ambulating for the first 3 months postoperatively. Outpatient physical therapy is typically started 2 weeks after surgery, and the patient is taught exercise programs to improve core muscle strength and function.

3.3.6 Management of complications

Our patients tolerate this MI-TLIF procedure exceptionally well. Potential perioperative complications include infection, hematoma, hardware malposition or failure, neurological injury, and cerebrospinal fluid leakage. Perioperative antibiotics, meticulous wound closure, and appropriate dressing changes can prevent wound infections. Proper utilization of fluoroscopic imaging and stimulation of K-wires and pedicle screws minimize the risk of instrumentation malposition and nerve root impingement. A small durotomy can be successfully treated with Gelfoam to cover the defect, followed by fibrin glue, followed by meticulous wound closure using a running locking nylon stitch. Complications can be limited by adequate surgical training and critical patient selection. Most postoperative would infections are superficial and above the fascial plane and can be treated with a week's course of oral antibiotics.

4. Clinical series

Using this technique, the following represents our MI-TLIF clinical series comprised 405 consecutive cases. The clinical characteristics are seen in **Table 2**. The average age of patients in the series was 64 years with most being female (60%). Forty-five percent of patients were classified as obese. The primary condition was treated with spondylolisthesis and spinal stenosis most commonly at the L4–5 level with back pain as the primary complaint. High blood pressure, diabetes, and high cholesterol were the most commonly seen co-morbidities.

Parameter	Patient data			
Age (years)	64.1 ± 12.5			
Sex (males:females%)	39.9%: 60.1%			
Symptoms duration	92.3 ± 16.5 months			
BMI categorization				
BMI less than or equal to 30 kg/m2	55.8%			
BMI 30.1–34.9 kg/m2 (Class I Obesity)	22.6%			
BMI 35.0–39.9 kg/m2 (Class II Obesity)	14.4%			
BMI ≥40.0 kg/m2 (Class III Obesity)	7.2%			
Diagnosis	**Total**	**L4/L5**	**L5/S1**	**L3/L4**
Spondylolisthesis	262 (65.1%)	28.03%	20.1%	16.9%
Spinal stenosis	261 (64.7%)	44.7%	11.2%	19.3%
Foraminal stenosis	226 (56.1%)	48.1%	20.3%	16.9%
Degenerative disk disease	95 (23.8%)	11.7%	11.4%	4.9%
Herniated disk	135 (33.5%)	6.9%	5.7%	1.2%
Synovial cyst	18 (4.4%)			
Degenerative scoliosis	149 (36.9%)			
Presenting symptoms				
Back pain	367 (91.1%)			
Neurogenic claudications	165 (40.9%)			
Leg pain	145 (35.9%)			

Parameter	Patient data
Others	80 (19.9%)
Comorbidity	**Patient data**
Hypertension	95 (23.6%)
Diabetes	62 (15.4%)
High cholesterol	33 (8.9%)
Cardiovascular disease	29 (7.2%)
Smoking	33 (8.9%)
Urinary incontinence	11 (2.7%)
Stroke history	12 (2.9%)
Osteoporosis	8 (1.9%)
Hypothyroidism	41 (10.2%)
Fibromyalgia	10 (2.5%)
Cancer	50 (12.4%)
Rheumatoid arthritis	11 (2.7%)

Table 2.
Patient characteristics (n = 405).

5. Minimally invasive TLIF series

Patients had a significant improvement in visual analog scores (VASs), Oswestry Disability Index (ODI), and Short Form-36 (SF36) over the 5-year follow-up period (**Table 3**, **Figure 9**).

ODI: Oswestry Disability Index, VAS: visual analog scale, SF: Short Form, PhF: physical function, RLPh: role limitation due to physical health problem, RLE: role limitation due to emotional health problem.

Complication rates in these series were low with cerebrospinal fluid (CSF) leak/dural tear experienced in only 0.5% of patients. Fusion rates based on the Bridwell

Parameter.							
	Preop	Postop 3 mon	Postop 1 year	Postop 2 years	Postop 3 years	Postop 4 years	Postop 5 years
ODI	45.9 ± 16.4	29.3 ± 19.3	21.9 ± 17.8	25.9 ± 15.6	24.6 ± 18.9	24.7 ± 13.7	22.3 ± 17.6
P		0.0002	0.0001	0.047	0.015	0.008	0.012
VAS	6.9 ± 2.2	3.1 ± 2.2	2.3 ± 1.9	2.7 ± 1.8	2.2 ± 1.4	1.3 ± 1.5	2.8 ± 1.6
P		0.0001	0.0001	0.0082	0.0001	0.0001	0.0026
PhF	17.5 ± 11.9	62 ± 20.3	58.4 ± 26.5	56.8 ± 27.2	50.5 ± 26.7	66.9 ± 18.5	83.3 ± 10.3
P		0.13	*0.17*	0.03	0.21	*0.003*	*0.003*
RLPh	9 ± 10.3	53.7 ± 26.6	53.9 ± 31.7	59.4 ± 30.7	59.4 ± 24.7	67.3 ± 23.4	75 ± 22
P		0.046	*0.007*	0.002	0.025	*0.025*	*0.026*
RLE	43.7 ± 4.1	85.8 ± 19.5	85.9 ± 15.4	96.9 ± 4.2	65.8 ± 31.04	76.65 ± 25.2	87.5 ± 19.5
P		0.019	*0.08*	0.0002	0.36	*0.03*	*0.03*

Table 3.
VAS, ODI, and SF36 (v2) scores (5-year follow-up).

VAS, ODI, SF36(v2): 5 Years Follow Up

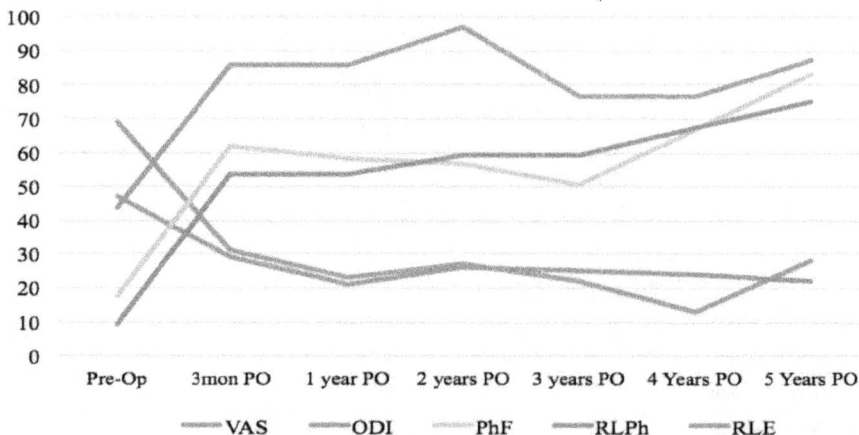

Figure 9.
Line graph demonstrating mean VAS of back pain, ODI and SF36 (v2) scores over 5 years follow up time. PhF: Physical function, RLPh: Role limitation due to physical health problem, RLE: Role limitation due to emotional health problem. PO: Post-operative. Op: Operative.

fusion criteria was extremely high with 97% achieving Grade I (**Table 4**). This was felt to be in large part because of the novel method of injecting the patient's own drilled morselized autograph into the properly prepared disk interspace. With loading of the filled disk space autograph bone material, according to Wolff's law, very high fusion rates can be achieved.

Postoperative complications	Neurological (<3 Months)	Non-neurological (%)
PO pain	2.9%	—
PO weakness	0.3%	—
Neurological PO deficit	0.5	—
Diaphragm injury	—	0.3%
Dysphagia	—	0.5%
Malpositioned screws	—	0.5%
Pulmonary embolism/thrombosis	—	0.7%
Ileus	—	1.2%
Wound problem (infection/hematoma)	0.9%	
Arrested	—	0.3%
Bone graft and cage	—	0.3%
CSF leak/dural tear	—	0.5%
Postoperative fusion rates11		
Description	**Grades**	**Percentage**
Fusion with remodeling and trabeculae	I	97.3%
Graft intact, not fully remodeled, no radiolucencies	II	1.7%
Graft intact, but a definite lucency	III	1%
Definitely not fused, collapsed	IV	—

PO: postoperative, CSF: cerebrospinal fluid.

Table 4.
Postoperative complications and fusion rates %, (n = 405).

6. Complication rates in minimally invasive TLIF series

Based on monthly recorded morbidity and mortality data, complications rates in this series were extremely low (**Figure 10**).

Post-Op 5 Years Morbidity and Mortality

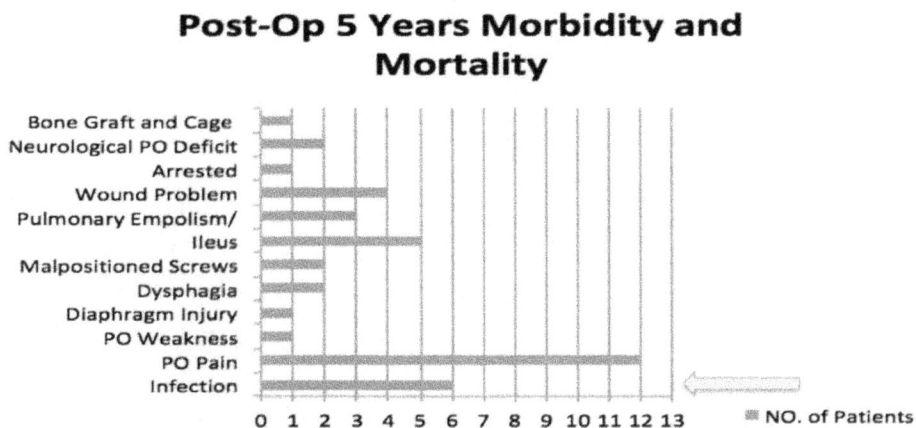

Figure 10.
Morbidity and mortality: 5-year follow-up.

7. Conclusion

The novel MI-TLIF approach and technology reviewed in this chapter afford significant short- and long-term improvements for patients suffering from debilitating low back pain. Long-term benefits include a reduced rate of adjacent segment disease requiring reoperation, high rates of fusion, and low complication rates. Clinically, our patients have been extremely satisfied in the treatment of their chronic back pain disorders. The majority of our patients are completely pain-free and have returned to work full time and are able to resume activities of daily living.

Conflict of interest

Thompson MIS/BoneBac: Stock Ownership, Orthofix: Speaker Bureau, Thieme Publishing Inc.: Royalties.

Author details

Mick Perez-Cruet[1,2]*, Ramiro Pérez de la Torre[2] and Siddharth Ramanathan[1]

1 Department of Neurosurgery, Oakland University William Beaumont, School of Medicine, Rochester, MI, United States

2 Department of Neurosurgery, Michigan Head and Spine Institute, Royal Oak, MI, United States

*Address all correspondence to: perezcruet@yahoo.com

IntechOpen

References

[1] Allain J, Dufour T. Anterior lumbar fusion techniques: ALIF, OLIF, DLIF, LLIF, IXLIF. Orthopaedics & Traumatology, Surgery & Research. 2020;**106**(1S):S149-S157

[2] Patel D, Yoo J, Karmakar S, Lamoutte E, Singh K. Interbody options in lumbar fusion. Spine Surgery. 2019;**5**(Suppl. 1):S19-S24

[3] Choudri T, Mummaneni P, Dhall S, Eck J, Groff M, Ghogawala Z, et al. Guideline update for the performance of fusion procedures for degenerative disease of the lumbar spine. Part 4: Radiographic assessment of fusion status. Journal of Neurosurgery. Spine. 2014;**21**(1):23-30

[4] Babu MA, Coumans JV, Carter BS, Taylor WR, Kasper EM, Roitberg BZ, et al. A review of lumbar spinal instrumentation: Evidence and controversy. Journal of Neurology, Neurosurgery, and Psychiatry. 2011;**82**(9):948-951

[5] Yoshihara H. Surgical options for lumbosacral fusion: Biomechanical stability, advantage, disadvantage and affecting factors in selecting options. European Journal of Orthopaedic Surgery and Traumatology. 2014; **24**(Suppl. 1):S73-S82

[6] Kerolus M, Turel MK, Tan L, Deutsch H. Stand-alone anterior lumbar interbody fusion: Indications, techniques, surgical outcomes and complications. Expert Review of Medical Devices. 2016;**13**(12):1127-1136

[7] de la Torre RA P, Kelkar PS, Beier A, et al. Decompression, transforaminal lumbar interbody fusion, reduction, and percutaneous pedicle screw fixation. In: Perez-Cruet MJ, Beisse RW, Pimenta L, Kim DH, editors. Minimally Invasive Spine Fusion: Techniques and Operative Nuances. St. Louis: Quality Medical Publishing; 2011. pp. 345-367

[8] Perez-Cruet MJ, Hussain NS, White GZ, Begun EM, Collins RA, Fahim DK, et al. Quality-of-life outcomes with minimally invasive Transforaminal lumbar interbody fusion based on long-term analysis of 304 consecutive patients. Spine. 2014;**39**(3):E191-E198

[9] Khechen B, Haws BE, Patel DV, Narain AS, Hijji FY, Guntin JA, et al. Comparison of postoperative outcomes between primary MIS TLIF and MIS TLIF with revision decompression. Spine (Phila Pa 1976). 2019;**44**(2): 150-156

[10] Teng I, Han J, Phan K, Mobbs R. A meta-analysis comparing ALIF, PLIF, TLIF and LLIF. Journal of Clinical Neuroscience. 2017;**44**:11-17

[11] Hammad A, Wirries A, Ardeshiri A, Nikiforov O, Geiger F. Open versus minimally invasive TLIF: Literature review and meta-analysis. Journal of Orthopaedic Surgery and Research. 2019;**14**(1):229

[12] Garg B, Mehta N. Minimally invasive transforaminal lumbar interbody fusion (MI-TLIF): A review of indications, technique, results and complications. Journal of Clinical Orthopaedics & Trauma. 2019;**10** (Suppl. 1):S156-S162

[13] Momin A, Steinmetz M. Evolution of minimally invasive lumbar spine surgery. World Neurosurgery. 2020;**140**:622-626

[14] Mummaneni P, Bisson E, Kerezoudis P, Glassman S, Foley K, Slotkin J, et al. Minimally invasive versus open fusion for grade I degenerative lumbar spondylolisthesis: Analysis of the quality. Neurosurgical Focus. 2017;**43**(2):E11 Outcomes Database

[15] Ghogawala Z, Dziura J, Butler WE, Dai F, Terrin N, Magge SN, et al.

Laminectomy plus fusion versus laminectomy alone for lumbar spondylolisthesis. The New England Journal of Medicine. April 14, 2016;**374**(15):1424-1434

[16] Wang B, Hua W, Ke W, Lu S, Li X, Zeng X, et al. Biomechanical evaluation of Transforaminal lumbar interbody fusion and oblique lumbar interbody fusion on the adjacent segment: A finite element analysis. World Neurosurgery. 2019;**126**:e819-e824

[17] Villavicencio A, Nurneikiene S, Roeca C, Nelson L, Mason A. Minimally invasive versus open transforaminal lumbar interbody fusion. Surgical Neurology International. 2010;**1**:12

[18] Habib A, Smith ZA, Lawton CD. Fessler RG minimally invasive transforaminal lumbar interbody busion: A perspective on current evidence and clinical knowledge. Minim Invasive Surgery. 2012;**2012**:657342

[19] Scheufler KM, Dohmen H, Vougioukas VI. Percutaneous transforaminal lumbar interbody fusion for the treatment of degenerative lumbar instability. Neurosurgery. 2007;**60**(4, suppl. 2):203-212

[20] Dhall SS, Wang MY, Mummaneni PV. Clinical and radiographic comparison of mini-open transforaminal lumbar interbody fusion with open transforaminal lumbar interbody fusion in 42 patients with long-term follow-up: Clinical article. Journal of Neurosurgery: Spine. 2008;**9**(6):560-565

[21] Peng CWB, Yue WM, Poh SY, Yeo W, Tan SB. Clinical and radiological outcomes of minimally invasive versus open transforaminal lumbar interbody fusion. Spine. 2009;**34**(13):1385-1389

[22] Schizas C, Tzinieris N, Tsiridis E, Kosmopoulos V. Minimally invasive versus open transforaminal lumbar

interbody fusion: Evaluating initial experience. International Orthopaedics. 2009;**33**(6):1683-1688

[23] Wang J, Zhou Y, Zhang ZF, Li CQ, Zheng WJ, Liu J. Comparison of one-level minimally invasive and open transforaminal lumbar interbody fusion in degenerative and isthmic spondylolisthesis grades 1 and 2. European Spine Journal. 2010;**19**(10):1780-1784

[24] Champagne P, Walsh C, Diabira J, Plante M, Wang Z, Boubez G, et al. Sagittal balance correction following lumbar interbody fusion: A comparison of the three approaches. Asian Spine Journal. 2019;**13**(3):450-458

[25] Mobbs R, Phan K, Malham G, Seex K, Rao P. Lumbar interbody fusion: Techniques, indications and comparison of interbody fusion options including PLIF, TLIF, MI-TLIF, OLIF/ATP, LLIF and ALIF. Journal of Spine Surgery. 2015;**1**(1):2-18

[26] Terman SW, Yee TJ, Lau D, Khan AA, La Marca F, Park P. Minimally invasive versus open transforaminal lumbar interbody fusion: Comparison of clinical outcomes among obese patients. Journal of Neurosurgery Spine. June 2014;**20**(6):644-652. DOI: 10.3171/2014.2.SPINE13794. [Epub Apr 18, 2014]

[27] Xi MA, Tong HC, Fahim DK, Perez-Cruet M. Using provocative discography and computed tomography to select patients with refractory discogenic low back pain for lumbar fusion surgery. Cureus. Feb 27, 2016;**8**(2):e514

[28] Staub BN, Sadrameli SS. The use of robotics in minimally invasive spine surgery. Journal of Spine Surgery. 2019;**5**(Suppl. 1):S31-S40

[29] Vo CD, Jiang B, Azad TD, Crawford NR, Bydon A. Theodore N robotic spine surgery: Current state in

minimally invasive surgery. Global
Spine Journal. 2020;**10**(Suppl. 2):
34S-40S

[30] Sears WR, Sergides IG, Kazemi N,
Smith M, White GJ, Osburg B. Incidence
and prevalence of surgery at segments
adjacent to a previous posterior lumbar
arthrodesis. The Spine Journal.
2011;**11**:11-20

Minimally Invasive Treatment of Spinal Malignancy

Chapter 11

Minimally Invasive Treatment of Spinal Metastasis

Eric R. Mong and Daniel K. Fahim

Abstract

Advancements in the treatment of systemic cancer have improved life expectancy in cancer patients and consequently the incidence of spinal metastasis. Traditionally, open spinal approaches combined with cEBRT (conventional external beam radiation therapy) allowed for local tumor control as well as stabilization and decompression of the spine and neural elements, but these larger operations can be fraught with one complications and delayed healing as well as additional morbidity. Recently, minimally invasive spine techniques are becoming increasingly popular in the treatment of spinal metastasis for many reasons, including smaller incisions with less perioperative complications and potential for expedited time to radiation therapy. These techniques include kyphoplasty with radiofrequency ablation, percutaneous stabilization, laminectomy, and epidural tumor resection through tubular retractors, as well as minimally invasive corpectomy. These techniques combined with highly conformal stereotactic radiosurgery have led to the advent of separation surgery, which allows for decompression of neural elements while creating space between neural elements and the tumor so adequate radiation may be delivered, improving local tumor control. The versatility of these minimally invasive techniques has significantly improved the modern management of metastatic disease of the spine by protecting and restoring the patient's quality of life while allowing them to quickly resume radiation and systemic treatment.

Keywords: minimally invasive spine, spinal tumors, spinal metastasis, separation surgery, spinal stabilization

1. Introduction

The spine is the most common site of bony metastases [1]. Significant improvements in treatment modalities in the form of chemotherapy, immunotherapy, and radiation therapy have led to increased life expectancy for cancer patients [2]. Consequently, the incidence of metastatic cancer has been increasing. Twenty to seventy percent of patients with metastatic cancer are expected to develop spinal metastases during the course of their disease [3, 4]. The increased incidence of spinal metastases has increased the need for surgical treatment of its complications including symptomatic cord compression and mechanical instability. The goal of neurosurgical treatment includes addressing mechanical instability, correcting deformity, halting or reversing neurologic deficit, and improving pain and quality of life [5]. Traditionally, open surgical approaches have been used for surgical management of spinal metastatic disease. Through the advances made in minimally invasive spine surgery (MISS) for trauma and deformity, MISS for tumors is becoming more common due to decreased perioperative morbidity in cancer patients with similar efficacy to traditional open approaches.

2. Evaluation of patients with spinal metastases

Patients with metastatic spinal cancer often have significant comorbidities and complex clinical scenarios that require multidisciplinary evaluation and treatment. The NOMS (neurologic, oncologic, mechanical, systemic) framework, developed at the Memorial Sloan-Kettering Cancer Center, assesses neurologic, oncologic, mechanical, and systemic factors during the decision-making process for the treatment of spinal tumors across multiple specialties. The oncologic factors include the predicted responses and durability of available treatment modalities including chemotherapy, immunotherapy, and radiotherapy [5, 6]. The systemic consideration predicts both the patient's ability to tolerate multimodal treatments and overall survival based on the grade and stage of disease as well as the overall health of the patient [5]. The neurologic and mechanical criteria are of particular interest to the neurosurgeon involved in the patient's care.

The neurologic component of the NOMS framework assesses the presence of myelopathy or radiculopathy and is related to epidural compression of the spinal cord and nerve roots. It is estimated that symptomatic cord compression occurs in up to 20% of patients with metastatic cancer and may be the initial symptom in 5–10% [7, 8]. Cord compression above the conus may present with myelopathy, weakness, numbness, urinary urgency. Below the level of the conus, compression of the cauda equina may present with lower motor neuron symptoms of unilateral or bilateral motor weakness, radiculopathy, numbness, or urinary retention. Such symptoms require urgent neurosurgical intervention to either stabilize or improve neurologic function.

The mechanical criteria concerns the stability of the vertebral column affected by metastatic tumor and can be further analyzed by the SINS (spinal instability neoplastic score) criteria [9]. The SINS criteria assess the location of the spine affected including junctional areas, the presence of mechanical pain, type of bony lesions, spinal alignment, amount of vertebral body collapse, and posterolateral involvement [9]. Scores of 0–6 are deemed stable, whereas 7–12 are indeterminate but suggest the possibility of instability, 13–18 are unstable. SINS scores of 7–18 warrant neurosurgical consultation. Overall, the sensitivity and specificity of the SINS criteria for potentially unstable and unstable spinal lesions are 95.7% and 79.5%, respectively [9].

3. Traditional/open operative intervention

Historically, symptomatic metastatic spine disease has been treated with open surgical approaches. Traditional open approaches provide adequate visualization of tumor as well as spinal anatomy. The wide exposures allow for sufficient decompression of the spinal cord and nerve roots, stabilization for mechanical instability, and the opportunity for gross total resection, if indicated. However, the larger incisions with open approaches often lead to prolonged wound healing, which may delay postoperative chemotherapy and radiation. Larger surgical incisions also involve greater blood loss, which is concerning given the high rate of bone marrow toxicity and anemia in metastatic cancer patients, essentially all of whom exhibit preoperative anemia. Larger incisions also have higher incidence of wound breakdown and infections. Greater tissue damage contributes to greater postoperative pain, opioid requirements, and poor quality of life in patients with limited life expectancy.

4. The evolving role of MISS

The advent of MISS techniques, initially for the treatment of degenerative conditions followed by applications in trauma, has led to the adoption of these techniques for oncological disease of the spine as well. MISS offers the opportunity to treat mechanical instability and epidural spinal compression in patients who otherwise may not tolerate a more extensive surgical approach due to heavy systemic disease burden [4, 10]. When considering the need for radiation and systemic chemotherapy, one postoperative barrier to adjuvant treatment is proper healing of the surgical incision. Smaller incisions involved with minimally invasive approaches may offer expedited time to chemotherapy and radiation therapy [4].

Many benefits of MISS can be attributed to minimizing tissue damage. Less tissue damage may also allow for quicker pain relief, decreased intake of opioids during the postoperative period, which may translate to early mobilization, functional recovery, and improvement in quality of life [4, 11]. Smaller incisions are also associated with less perioperative blood loss and transfusion requirements [12, 13].

Other benefits of MISS include preservation of the posterior elements, including the multifidus, which is one of the largest contributors of the posterior tension band and overall stabilization of the spine [14]. Given that many patients with spinal metastases frequently have compromised integrity of the spine, preservation of the tension band may prevent postoperative instability, kyphosis, and forms of instrumentation failure including screw pullout [14].

Disadvantages of MISS techniques include difficulty recognizing microsurgical anatomy given distortion by pathology in smaller spaces, as well as highly vascularized pathology that may lead to bleeding that is difficult to control. Both of these difficulties may require conversion to open approach [15]. Furthermore, the intricacy involved with MISS may lead to longer operative times [15]. Despite these risks, the ability for MISS techniques to offer preservation of function, symptomatic and palliative treatment for metastatic cancer with lower perioperative morbidity remains of great interest.

5. Evolving role of radiation

Both cEBRT (conventional external beam radiation therapy) and SBRT (stereotactic body radiation therapy) and SRS (stereotactic radiosurgery) have been heavily involved in the treatment of MESCC (metastatic epidural spinal cord compression). Historically, palliative radiation in the form of cEBRT was used and has been shown to have stronger outcomes in pain relief, neurologic status, and local control in patients with radiosensitive tumors compared with radioresistant tumors [16, 17]. Additionally, the rate of local control was found to be inversely proportional to tumor size for patients undergoing cEBRT [18]. The advent of SRS and SBRT has significantly improved the treatment of MESCC by its ability to deliver high doses of radiation to smaller targets, minimizing damage to adjacent neurologic structures (**Figure 1**). Compared with cEBRT, SRS is able to provide local control independent of tumor histology [19]. Tumor recurrence in patients that have undergone SRS has been shown to be dependent on the amount of radiation delivered rather than radiosensitivity of the tumor [5]. Furthermore, for patients undergoing epidural spine decompression followed by SBRT, the majority of tumor

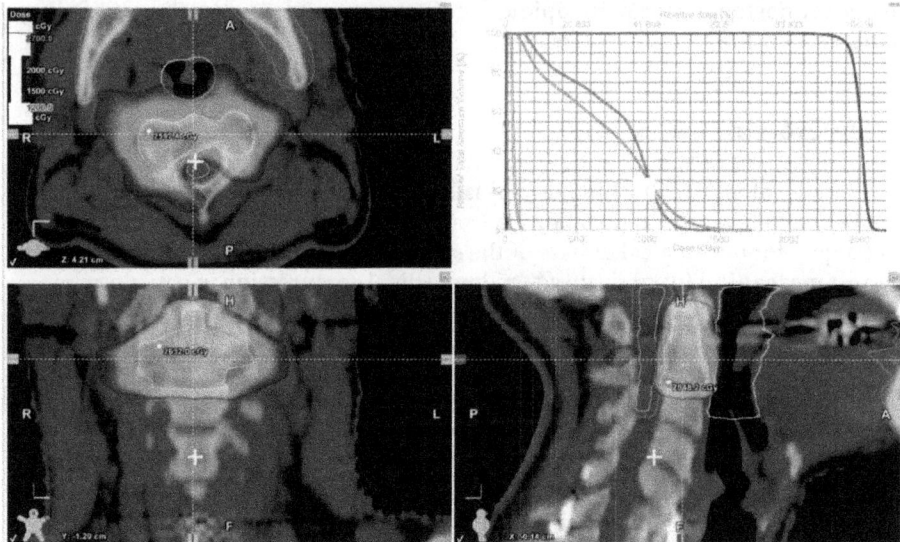

Figure 1.
(A) Axial, (B) coronal, (C) sagittal images showing a highly conformal stereotactic radiosurgery treatment plan to a C2 metastatic lesion secondary to thyroid cancer. The isodose lines can be seen around C2 and the structures at risk are also outlined (the oropharynx and upper esophagus in green and the spinal canal in purple). (D) Shows the relative isodose lines in graphic form, with the tumor dose curve on the far right and the overlapping green and purple dose curves in the middle of the graph representing the dose to the oropharynx and spinal canal, respectively.

recurrence arose from the portion of the tumor in the epidural space adjacent to the spinal cord that invariably receives an inadequate dose, due to the need to protect the neural structures from the potential damage of radiation [18, 20, 21]. Clearly, the benefits of radiation therapy must be balanced against the risks of damaging normal tissue.

6. Advent and benefits to separation surgery

It has been well established that radiation therapy is highly effective for local tumor control. A landmark study by Patchell et al. showed that direct decompressive surgery followed by conventional radiation for symptomatic epidural cord compression was superior to radiation alone [22]. This finding established the essential role of surgery in the management of MESCC. At the same time, advances in stereotactic radiosurgery made radiation alone an attractive alternative to surgery once again. However, cord tolerance always constrains the dose of radiation delivered to the tumor close to the spinal cord, in order to avoid irreversible neurological damage (radiation myelopathy). Radiation failure and tumor recurrence of epidural metastatic disease most often occur adjacent to the spinal cord and dura mater, given this is where the radiation dose is limited to prevent injury to important neurological structures. Continued advancements in microsurgical and radiosurgery techniques have led to the advent of separation surgery, which has decreased the need for aggressive approaches for gross total resection [3, 8, 12, 21].

The goal of separation surgery is to create space between the neural elements and the tumor, so an adequate radiation dose can be delivered to the tumor. The surgical technique involves circumferential dissection around the dura to create an ablative target for SRS while preserving or restoring neurologic function and providing local tumor control [8, 21]. This strategy is most beneficial to radioresistant tumors such as metastatic renal cell carcinoma, melanoma, thyroid carcinoma, colorectal carcinoma as well as previously radiated tumors and may decrease surgical-related complications of gross total resection or en bloc resection [11, 23].

The shift toward separation surgery has allowed for the introduction of subtotal resection with tubular or expandable retractors through a minimally invasive approach [8, 12]. Furthermore, the small incisions associated with MIS approaches may allow for earlier radiation therapy [11]. The most common approach for separation surgery is the posterolateral approach, which allows for posterior instrumentation and stabilization as well as circumferential decompression [11, 24]. The use of tubular retractors with ventral decompression via a transpedicular approach is growing in popularity [8]. Surgical access from a tubular retractor has the ability to create enough space ventral to the dura to allow for delivery of an adequate dose of radiation without harming the neural structures. This less invasive technique is also associated with a relatively low rate of hardware failure. Amankulor cited 2.8% incidence of hardware failure that may be associated with inadequate reconstruction of the anterior column following minimally invasive tumor debulking [25].

7. Laser interstitial therapy

Laser interstitial thermal therapy is an alternative method for treatment of epidural cord compression that may be performed via a percutaneous minimally invasive approach. This technique may achieve both epidural decompression and local control when combined with radiosurgery with less morbidity than surgery [26]. However, the time it takes for the tumor to respond to the treatment and shrink away may preclude widespread adoption of this technique. Compared with open decompression, there may be shorter interval to resume systemic treatment averaging 7.8 days [26]. Small, early studies suggest noninferiority of laser interstitial thermal therapy plus XRT compared with open decompression plus XRT in select patients [26].

8. MISS techniques for treating mechanical instability

Metastatic disease to the vertebral column requires assessment for mechanical instability via the SINS criteria. SINS score of 7–12 signifies potential instability and may require bracing, kyphoplasty, percutaneous stabilization, or a combination of the three. Higher SINS scores involve more serious deformity including translation, significant vertebral body collapse, and bilateral pedicle involvement, which require more extensive approaches including vertebrectomy with instrumentation.

8.1 Vertebral augmentation

Compression fractures of the anterior column and combination of anterior and middle columns with preservation of the posterior elements are amenable to percutaneous kyphoplasty. High-level evidence supports kyphoplasty and vertebroplasty as highly effective for stabilizing symptomatic pathologic compression fractures [12, 27, 44] and may be done via an extrapedicular or transpedicular approach. Kyphoplasty may be combined with radiofrequency ablation and biopsy, which allows for diagnosis as well as oncological treatment (**Figure 2**). Minimal incision provides the ability for expedited recovery without interruption of radiation and chemotherapy. Patients often experience improvement in pain and functional status after these minimally invasive outpatient procedures [14].

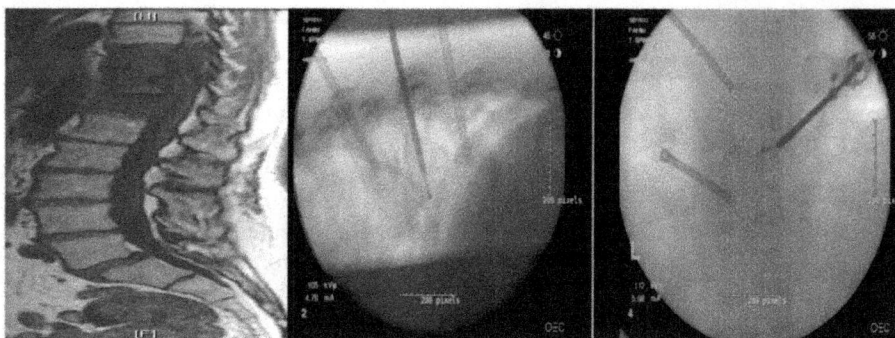

Figure 2.
(A) MRI shows multiple painful metastatic lesions at T10, T11, T12 despite treatment with fractionated radiation. (B) Lateral and (C) AP intraoperative images showing pedicle cannulation at all three levels and radiofrequency ablation probe in position of the T11 level.

8.2 Percutaneous stabilization

Indications for percutaneous stabilization include mechanical instability or as an adjunct to a decompressive surgery for neurologic deficit [10]. Instability is an indication for surgical stabilization regardless of radiosensitivity of the tumor [10, 23]. Percutaneous instrumentation can be performed via MISS or mini open approach over the levels of interest. MISS and mini-open approaches share the advantages of quicker healing time, decreased pain, and the potential for expedited time to administration of chemotherapy and radiation [28].

When considering components of the SINS criteria, compression fractures in junctional areas, as well as fractures with more than 50% loss in height, are subject to additional mechanical stress that may exacerbate fracture, deformity, and mechanical pain. These lesions may benefit from kyphoplasty with additional percutaneous stabilization. Furthermore, compression fractures with involvement of the posterior elements benefit from percutaneous stabilization and kyphoplasty. Burst fractures with significant retropulsion may require decompression with percutaneous stabilization.

Many cancer patients are predisposed to instrument-related complications given the metastatic nature of vertebral bodies combined with osteoporosis from systemic steroids and prior radiation. Combining fenestrated screws and cement augmentation with shorter constructs may lessen the cantilever effect on the spine and reduce incidence of screw pullout or pedicle fracture and proximal junctional kyphosis [12, 29, 30].

Patients with spinal instability and limited life expectancy may undergo percutaneous fixation without fusion. Silva and colleagues conducted a multicenter retrospective study that observed low implant failure rate in short and medium term without fusion [31]. Percutaneous screws may at times be placed with chemotherapeutic agents in attempt to reduce tumor size prior to resection. A case report describes the use of percutaneous screw stabilization with denosumab 6 months prior to en bloc spondylectomy for a spinal giant cell tumor associated with instability [32]. The tumor shrunk during this period, allowing for easier resection. This may be a consideration for a primary bone tumor, which requires aggressive total resection.

8.3 MISS decompression

Primary indications for surgical decompression of spinal metastasis are cord compression from radioresistant tumors as well as mechanical radiculopathy that can be localized to nerve root compression on imaging studies [6].

Tubular retractors may be used primarily for decompression of the posterior elements, but may also be used for ventral decompression as well as lateral decompression.

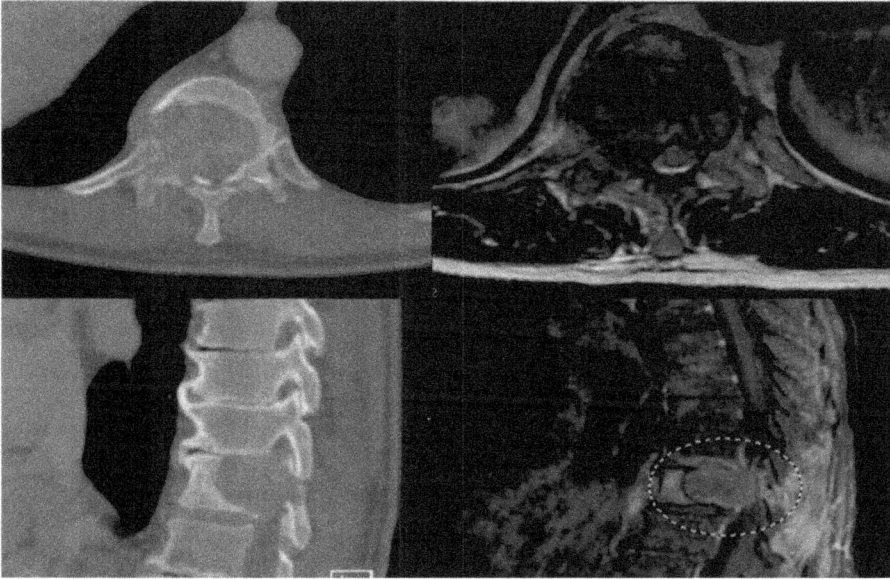

Figure 3.
Patient presenting with worsening back pain lower extremity paresthesias. (A) CT axial (B) CT showing lytic lesion with three column involvement, including unilateral pedicle involvement. (C) T1 MRI axial precontrast and T1 MRI sagittal post contrast shows epidural compression. Patient underwent thoracic laminectomy with unilateral transpedicular corpectomy with percutaneous stabilization two levels above and below the affected vertebrae.

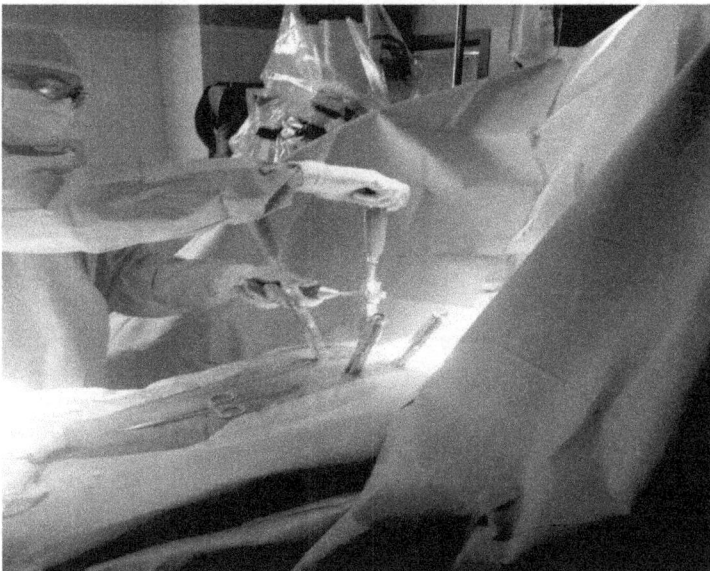

Figure 4.
MIS percutaneous screws and expandable retractor system for a unilateral transpedicular corpectomy.

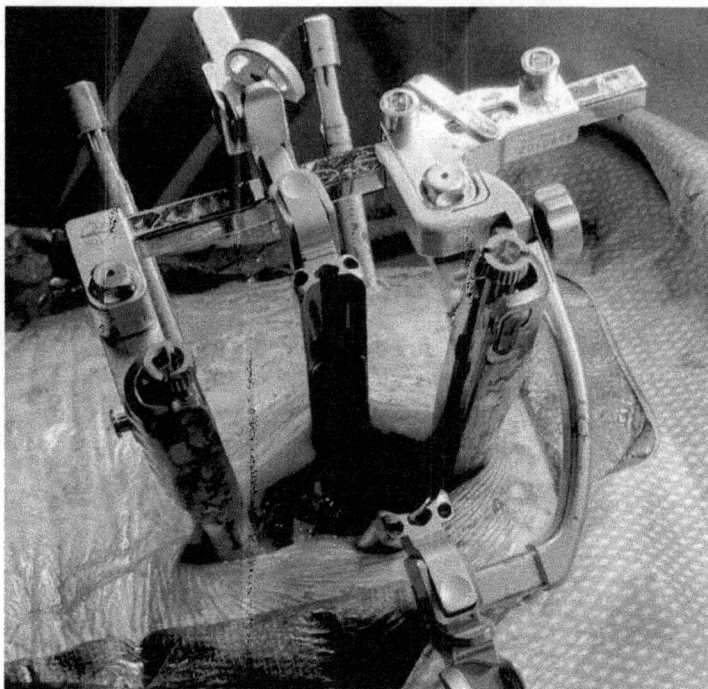

Figure 5.
Some expandable retractor systems used in minimally invasive unilateral decompression may be attached to the spinal fixation system used for percutaneous pedicle screw placement. Pictured is the space-D© retractor system by Medtronic.

8.4 Corpectomy with stabilization

Higher-grade SINS criteria involve significant vertebral body and posterior element compromise, which may require corpectomy with stabilization.

Mini-open and MIS approaches have been described for corpectomy with vertebral reconstruction. Such approaches are not as commonly utilized compared with the open approach. The open approach is often met with high morbidity, which has the potential to be especially detrimental to a cancer patient. A retrospective analysis of cohort of 49 adult patients with thoracic metastasis conducted by Lau et al. showed miniopen approach for thoracic transpedicular corpectomy with instrumentation had significantly less blood loss and hospital stay with no significant difference in complications or ASIA grade compared with the traditional open approach [33].

Extension of metastatic disease into pedicle or facet can cause mechanical radiculopathy as well as further destabilization of the spinal column [34]. If the lesion involves the anterior and middle columns and one pedicle, then unilateral approach tubular or expandable retractor may be used (**Figures 3–5**). If more extensive disease involves both pedicles, then bilateral tubular or expandable retractors can be used.

9. Expanding role of MISS management of spine tumors

There is essentially no role for MISS in primary vertebral body tumors, which require an en bloc spondylectomy for wide marginal resection [35]. There are multiple reports of both expandable and nonexpendable tubular retractors [36, 37] for extra-dural intraforaminal and intradural extramedullary tumors. Most reports use MISS techniques on lesions that span no more than two vertebral levels [38]. Combined approaches with tubular retractors have also be described to resect thoracic dumbbell-shaped ganglioneuroma in which tubular retractors were used for intraspinal component and robotic-assisted thoracoscopic resection for the extraforaminal intrathoracic component [39].

An interlaminar approach has been described for resection of intradural extramedullary lesions in the lumbar spine. With this technique, the pathology is approached through the center of the interlaminar space, where the space is the largest. This paramedian, bone-sparing approach theoretically preserves the posterior tension band and decreases postoperative instability [40].

Additionally, reports of flexible endoscopes via mini open incisions have been reported for the resection of intradural schwannomas at the cauda equine [41]. UT southwestern reports using a flexible endoscope through a minimal durotomy for aspiration of a dermoid tumor that spanned from T10-sacrum leading to functional recovery and remained asymptotic at 3 years despite small recurrence [42].

In general, treatment of intramedullary spinal cord tumors is associated with high neurologic morbidity. Given the need for GTR (gross total resection) in many of these tumors compared with metastatic tumors, which may undergo STR with separation surgery, GTR cannot be sacrificed for the previously mentioned benefits of MISS. A review of keyhole approaches for intradural tumors showed that only 5.3% of intramedullary lesions could be accessed [41]. MIS management of intra-medullary tumors is limited to mini open approach with hemilaminectomy and laminotomy for which GTR may still be achieved with benefit of smaller incision and preservation of vertebral stability [41, 42]. A retrospective study by Kahyaoglu et al., who treated 168 intramedullary tumors via hemilaminectomy, showed that neurologic complications increased when intramedullary tumors extended greater than three spinal segments, especially in thoracic spine compared with the cervical spine [43].

10. Conclusion

Advances in minimally invasive spine surgery techniques and concomitant advances in highly conformal stereotactic radiosurgery capabilities have revolution-ized the approach to symptomatic metastatic disease involving the spine. The role of surgery is to create a safe distance between the tumor and the neural structures for the safe delivery of a tumoricidal radiation dose and to treat mechanical instabil-ity of the spine. Versatility in the use of MISS techniques is essential for the modern management of metastatic disease of the spine to protect and restore the patient's quality of life and allow them to resume radiation and systemic treatment when indicated.

Author details

Eric R. Mong[1] and Daniel K. Fahim[1,2,3*]

1 Department of Neurosurgery, Beaumont Health, Southfield, MI, United States

2 Department of Neurosurgery, Oakland University William Beaumont School of Medicine, Auburn Hills, MI, United States

3 Michigan Head and Spine Institute, Southfield, MI, United States

*Address all correspondence to: daniel.fahim@beaumont.edu

IntechOpen

References

[1] Maccauro G, Spinelli MS, Mauro S, Perisano C, Graci C, Rosa MA. Physiopathology of spine metastasis. International Journal of Surgical Oncology. 2011;**2011**:107969. DOI: 10.1155/2011/107969

[2] Wewel JT, O'Toole JE. Epidemiology of spinal cord and column tumors. Neuro-Oncology Practice. 2020;7(1): i5-i9

[3] Laufer I, Rubin DG, Lis E. The NOMS framework: Approach to the treatment of spinal metastatic tumors. Oncologist. Jun 2013;**18**(6):744-751. DOI:10.1634/theoncologist.2012-0293

[4] Colangeli S, Capanna R, Bandiera S, Ghermandi R, Girolami M, Parchi PD, et al. Is minimally-invasive spinal surgery a reliable treatment option in symptomatic spinal metastasis? European Review for Medical and Pharmacological Sciences. 2020; **24**(12):6526-6532

[5] Laufer I, Iorgulescu JB, Chapman T, et al. Local disease control for spinal metastases following "separation surgery" and adjuvant hypofractionated or high-dose single-fraction stereotactic radiosurgery: Outcome analysis in 186 patients. Journal of Neurosurgery. Spine. 2013;**18**:207-214

[6] Barzilai O, Boriani S, Fisher CG, et al. Essential concepts for the Management of Metastatic Spine Disease: What the surgeon should know and practice. Global The Spine Journal. May 2019;**9**(1 Suppl):98-107

[7] Miscusi M, Polli FM, Forcato S, Ricciardi L, Frati A, Cimatti M, et al. Comparison of minimally invasive surgery with standard open surgery for vertebral thoracic metastases causing acute myelopathy in patients with short- or mid-term life expectancy: Surgical technique and early clinical results. Journal of Neurosurgery. Spine. 2015;**22**(5):518-525

[8] De la Garza RR, Echt M, Gelfand Y, Yanamadala V, Yassari R. Minimally invasive tubular separation surgery for metastatic spinal cord compression: 2-dimensional operative video. Operative Neurosurgery. 2021; **20**(5):E356

[9] Fisher CG, DiPaola CP, Ryken TC, Bilsky MH, Shaffrey CI, Berven SH, et al. A novel classification system for spinal instability in neoplastic disease: An evidence-based approach and expert consensus from the spine oncology study group. Spine. 2010;**35**: E1221-E1229

[10] Zuckerman SL, Laufer I, Sahgal A, Yamada YJ, Schmidt MH, Chou D, et al. When less is more: The indications for MIS techniques and separation surgery in metastatic spine disease. Spine. 2016;**41**(Suppl. 20):S246-S253

[11] Turel MK, Kerolus MG, O'Toole JE. Minimally invasive "separation surgery" plus adjuvant stereotactic radiotherapy in the management of spinal epidural metastases. Journal of Craniovertebral Junction and Spine. 2017;**8**(2):119-126

[12] Barzilai O, Bilsky MH, Laufer I. The role of minimal access surgery in the treatment of spinal metastatic Tumors. Global Spine Journal. 2020;**10**(Suppl. 2): 79S-87S

[13] Pranata R, Lim MA, Vania R, Bagus Mahadewa TG. Minimal invasive surgery instrumented fusion versus conventional open surgical instrumented fusion for the treatment of spinal metastases: A systematic review and Meta-analysis. World Neurosurgery. 2021;**148**:e264-e274. DOI: 10.1016/j.wneu.2020.12.130

[14] Reinas R, Kitumba D, Pereira L, Alves OL. Minimally invasive surgery

for spinal fractures due to multiple myeloma. Journal of Craniovertebral Junction and Spine. 2021;**12**(2):117-122. DOI: 10.4103/jcvjs.jcvjs_2_21

[15] Morgen SS, Hansen LV, Karbo T, Svardal-Stelmer R, Gehrchen M, Dahl B. Minimal access *vs.* open spine surgery in patients with metastatic spinal cord compression - a one-Center randomized controlled trial. Anticancer Research. 2020;**40**(10):5673-5678. DOI: 10.21873/anticanres.114581

[16] Maranzano E, Latini P. Effectiveness of radiation therapy without surgery in metastatic spinal cord compression: Final results from a prospective trial. International Journal of Radiation Oncology, Biology, Physics. 1995;**32**(4):959-967

[17] Barzilai O, Fisher CG, Bilsky MH. State of the art treatment of spinal metastatic disease. Neurosurgery. 2018;**82**:757-769

[18] Cofano F, Di Perna G, Alberti A, Baldassarre BM, Ajello M, Marengo N, et al. Neurological outcomes after surgery for spinal metastases in symptomatic patients: Does the type of decompression play a role? A comparison between different strategies in a 10-year experience. Journal of Bone Oncology. 2020;**26**:100340

[19] Yamada Y, Bilsky MH, Lovelock DM, Venkatraman ES, Toner S, Johnson J, et al. High-dose, single-fraction image-guided intensity-modulated radiotherapy for metastatic spinal lesions. International Journal of Radiation Oncology, Biology, Physics. 2008;**71**(2):484-490

[20] Al-Omair A, Masucci L, Masson-Cote L, et al. Surgical resection of epidural disease improves local control following postoperative spine stereotactic body radiotherapy. Neuro-Oncology. 2013;**15**(10):1413-1419

[21] Di Perna G, Cofano F, Mantovani C, Badellino S, Marengo N, Ajello M, et al. Separation surgery for metastatic epidural spinal cord compression: A qualitative review. Journal of Bone Oncology. 2020;**25**:100320

[22] Patchell RA, Tibbs PA, Regine WF, Payne R, Saris S, Kryscio RJ, et al. Direct decompressive surgical resection in the treatment of spinal cord compression caused by metastatic cancer: A randomised trial. Lancet. 2005;**366**(9486):643-648

[23] Moussazadeh N, Rubin DG, McLaughlin L, et al. Short-segment percutaneous pedicle screw fixation with cement augmentation for tumor-induced spinal instability. The Spine Journal. 2015;**15**:1609-1617

[24] Saigal R, Wadhwa R, Mummaneni PV, Chou D. Minimally invasive extracavitary transpedicular corpectomy for the management of spinal tumors. Neurosurgery Clinics of North America. 2014 Apr;**25**(2):305-315. DOI: 10.1016/j.nec.2013.12.008

[25] Amankulor NM, Xu R, Iorgulescu JB, et al. The incidence and patterns of hardware failure after separation surgery in patients with spinal metastatic tumors. The Spine Journal. 2014;**14**:1850-1859

[26] de Almeida Bastos DC, Everson RG, de Oliveira Santos BF, Habib A, Vega RA, Oro M, et al. A comparison of spinal laser interstitial thermotherapy with open surgery for metastatic thoracic epidural spinal cord compression. Journal of Neurosurgery. Spine. Jan 2020;1-9

[27] Gaitanis IN, Hadjipavlou AG, Katonis PG, Tzermiadianos MN, Pasku DS, Patwardhan AG. Balloon kyphoplasty for the treatment of pathological vertebral compressive fractures. European Spine Journal. 2005;**14**(3):250-260

[28] Joseph JR, Spratt DE, Oppenlander ME, Park P, Szerlip NJ. Analysis of outcomes between traditional open versus Mini-open approach in surgical treatment of spinal metastasis. World Neurosurgery. 2019;**130**:e467-e474. DOI: 10.1016/j.wneu.2019.06.121

[29] Harel R, Doron O, Knoller N. Minimally invasive spine metastatic tumor resection and stabilization: New technology yield improved outcome. BioMed Research International. 2015;**2015**:948373. DOI: 10.1155/2015/948373

[30] Huangxs S, Christiansen PA, Tan H, Smith JS, Shaffrey ME, Uribe JS, et al. Mini-open lateral Corpectomy for thoracolumbar junction lesions. Operative Neurosurgery. 2020;**18**(6): 640-647

[31] Silva A, Yurac R, Guiroy A, Bravo O, Morales Ciancio A, Landriel F, et al. Low implant failure rate of percutaneous fixation for spinal metastases: A Multicenter retrospective study. World Neurosurgery. 2021;**148**:e627-e634. DOI: 10.1016/j.wneu.2021.01.047

[32] Minato K, Hirano T, Kawashima H, Yamagishi T, Watanabe K, Ohashi M, et al. Minimally invasive spinal stabilization with Denosumab before Total Spondylectomy for a collapsing lower lumbar spinal Giant cell tumor. Acta Medica Okayama. 2021;**75**(1):95-101

[33] Lau D, Chou D. Posterior thoracic corpectomy with cage reconstruction for metastatic spinal tumors: Comparing the mini-open approach to the open approach. Journal of Neurosurgery. Spine. 2015;**23**(2):217-227

[34] Moliterno J, Veselis CA, Hershey MA, Lis E, Laufer I, Bilsky MH. Improvement in pain after lumbar surgery in cancer patients with mechanical radiculopathy. The Spine Journal. 2014;**14**:2434-2439

[35] Liljenqvist U, Lerner T, Halm H, Buerger H, Gosheger G, Winkelmann W. En bloc spondylectomy in malignant tumors of the spine. European Spine Journal. 2008;**17**(4):600-609

[36] Nzokou A, Weil AG, Shedid D. Minimally invasive removal of thoracic and lumbar spinal tumors using a nonexpandable tubular retractor. Journal of Neurosurgery. Spine. 2013;**19**(6):708-715. DOI: 10.3171/2013.9.SPINE121061. Erratum in: Journal of Neurosurgery. Spine, 20(5), 602

[37] Soriano Sánchez JA, Soto García ME, Soriano Solís S, Rodríguez García M, Trejo Huerta P, Sánchez Escandón O, et al. Microsurgical resection of Intraspinal benign Tumors using non-Expansile tubular access. World Neurosurgery. 2020;**133**:e97-e104. DOI: 10.1016/j.wneu.2019.08.170

[38] Thavara BD, Kidangan GS, Rajagopalawarrier B. Analysis of the surgical technique and outcome of the thoracic and lumbar Intradural spinal tumor excision using minimally invasive tubular retractor system. Asian Journal of Neurosurgery. 2019;**14**(2): 453-460

[39] Wewel JT, Kasliwal MK, Chmielewski GW, O'Toole JE. Complete anterior-posterior minimally invasive thoracoscopic robotic-assisted and posterior tubular approach for resection of thoracic dumbbell tumor. Journal of Craniovertebral Junction and Spine. 2020;**11**(2):148-151

[40] Zhu YJ, Ying GY, Chen AQ, Wang LL, Yu DF, Zhu LL, et al. Minimally invasive removal of lumbar intradural extramedullary lesions using the interlaminar approach. Neurosurgical Focus. 2015;**39**(2):E10

[41] Mende KC, Krätzig T, Mohme M, Westphal M, Eicker SO. Keyhole approaches to intradural pathologies. Neurosurgical Focus. 2017;**43**(2):E5

[42] Hatchette CV, Aoun SG, El Ahmadieh TY, Smalley L, Patel AR, Zhao L, et al. Minimally invasive endoscopic aspiration of a spinal epidural Dermoid cyst extending from T10 to the sacrum: 2-dimensional operative video. Operative Neurosurgery. 2020;**18**(5):E172

[43] Yuce İ, Kahyaoğlu O, Çavuşoğlu HA, Ataseven M, Çavuşoğlu H, Aydın Y. Surgical treatment and outcomes of intramedullary tumors by minimally invasive approach. Journal of Clinical Neuroscience. 2021;**86**:26-31

[44] Sawakami K, Yamazaki A, Ishikawa S, et al. Polymethyl methacrylate augmentation of pedicle screws increases the initial fixation in osteoporotic spine patients. Journal of Spinal Disorders & Techniques. 2012;**25**:E28-E35

Chapter 12

Robotic Guided Minimally Invasive Spine Surgery

Ram Kiran Alluri, Ahilan Sivaganesan, Avani S. Vaishnav and Sheeraz A. Qureshi

Abstract

Minimally invasive spine surgery (MISS) continues to evolve, and the advent of robotic spine technology may play a role in further facilitating MISS techniques, increasing safety, and improving patient outcomes. In this chapter we review early limitations of spinal robotic systems and go over currently available spinal robotic systems. We then summarize the evidence-based advantages of robotic spine surgery, with an emphasis on pedicle screw placement. Additionally, we review some common and expanded clinical applications of robotic spine technology to facilitate MISS. The chapter concludes with a discussion regarding the current limitations and future directions of this relatively novel technology as it applies to MISS.

Keywords: minimally invasive spine surgery, robotic spine surgery, spinal robotics, minimally invasive surgery

1. Introduction

Spine surgery has continued to evolve over the past several decades and significant advancements have been made in operative techniques, biomaterials, implant design, and intraoperative imaging. Many of these advances have been catalyzed by the advent and progression of minimally invasive spine surgery (MISS). MISS allows for less muscle dissection, smaller incisions, decreased post-operative pain, faster recovery, and potentially improved functional outcomes [1–4]. While MISS has evolved from the time of its inception, in part due to advancements in retractors, instruments, and intraoperative imaging, the goals have remained the same: adequate decompression of neural elements with or without vertebral column stabilization, while minimizing soft tissue trauma.

The unique challenge of MISS is that accurate identification of complex three-dimensional landmarks, decompression, and instrumentation all rely substantially on intraoperative imaging, given that anatomic landmarks are often not easily visualized or palpable. The reliance on intraoperative imaging and the resultant occupational radiation exposure to the surgeon and perioperative staff during MISS has been met with concern [5–7], and has contributed to the limited adoption of MISS techniques by some surgeons [8].

Partly in response to these concerns, the use of real-time image guidance and navigation technologies - not dependent on traditional static fluoroscopic imaging - have rapidly evolved over the past two decades. So too have the clinical applications for robotic technology in MISS in an attempt to further improve accuracy, decrease complications, and improve patient-reported outcomes.

2. Robotic spine surgery

Robot-assisted surgery has been performed in multiple surgical sub-specialties including urology, gynecology, and general surgery. Spine surgeons, however, have been relatively late adopters of robotic technology. This may be due to the fact that spine procedures are often technically demanding and rely upon refined fine motor skills when working around neural and vascular elements, all of which can be even more challenging when utilizing small incisions and working corridors with MISS. However, robot-assisted MISS may play a role in allowing surgeons to improve manual dexterity, decrease tremors, and provide stability for instrumentation by providing a fixed working angle that increases accuracy and precision. While there are many purported benefits for robot-assisted spine surgery, many early attempts at integration of this technology into MISS were met with significant challenges.

Early problems with robot-assisted spine surgery involved errors in synchronization of intraoperative fluoroscopic images with preoperative three-dimensional (3D) imaging, deflection of the robotic arm resulting in decreased accuracy of navigation and instrumentation, challenges with the user interface, and software crashes [9]. One early study documented technical or clinical errors in over 50% of spine procedures performed using robotic assistance [10]. In the setting of these early challenges, the lack of initial clinical benefit, significant infrastructure cost, and a steep learning curve, widespread adoption was not initially seen for this potentially beneficial technology [11, 12]. Over recent years, however, the integration of 3D computer-assisted navigation, improvements in the software and user interface, and automation of the robotic arm have driven a resurgence of interest in the use of robotic technology in MISS.

Currently there are three United States (US) Food and Drug Administration (FDA) approved robots for spine surgery. The Mazor X (Medtronic Spine, Memphis, TN, USA) was launched commercially in 2016 and has recently been integrated with Stealth Navigation (Medtronic Navigation Louisville, CO, USA), which allows for real-time instrument tracking intraoperatively. The ExcelsiusGPS (Globus Medical, Inc., Audubon, PA, USA) launched in 2017 and was one of the first robotic spine systems with fully integrated navigation, also allowing for real-time instrument tracking. The ROSA Spine (Zimmer Biomet, Montpellier, France) is the third and final US FDA-approved robot to assist in spine surgery. It was originally approved in 2016, and a recent upgrade - the ROSA ONE - was approved in 2019. Compared to the previously mentioned robots, the ROSA platform allows for navigation and instrumentation across cranial, spine, and total knee arthroplasty procedures, making it a multi-purpose technology with hospital-wide applications. A fourth offering, the TiRobot (TINAVI Medical Technologies, Beijing, China), was approved in China as of 2016, and can also be used for other orthopedic applications outside of spine surgery.

3. Advantages of robotic spine surgery

In MISS, robotic technology is most commonly employed to place percutaneous pedicle screws without direct visualization of anatomic landmarks. The use of robot-assisted pedicle screw placement has been widely researched in terms of accuracy, proximal facet violation rates, radiation, operative time/efficiency, clinical outcomes, and complications as compared to traditional 2D fluoroscopic and 3D navigated pedicle screw placement.

3.1 Pedicle screw placement accuracy

Traditionally placed free-hand pedicle screws have relied on the identification of anatomic landmarks and intraoperative fluoroscopy. Misplaced screws can result in neurovascular complications, continued low back pain, and the potential for earlier-onset adjacent segment disease. In MISS surgery, the absence of directly visualized bony anatomy traditionally mandated even further reliance on fluoroscopic imaging, however 3D intraoperative real-time navigation has improved over the last decade and is readily available for most MISS procedures. While 3D navigation was a significant advancement in MISS, intraoperative navigation is not without its limitations, as it still relies upon surgeons' hand-eye coordination and focus, which can be compromised and fatigued with repetitive tasks (as is the case with multi-level fusion cases). The use of a robotic arm may allow for more accurate, precise, and reproducible pedicle screw placement by minimizing both human error and the mental/physical burden on surgeons [13, 14].

One of the first papers investigating the accuracy of robotic assisted pedicle screw placement demonstrated 91–98% accuracy depending on the plane assessed [15]. Since then, several studies have documented a 94–98% accuracy of pedicle screw placement with robotic systems [16–21]. Specifically comparing robotic-assisted to free-hand pedicle screw placement, two studies demonstrated significantly higher accuracy with robot-assisted placement [22, 23], and a third study demonstrated similar accuracy between the two pedicle screw techniques [21]. However, one prospective study did demonstrate decreased accuracy with robotic-assisted screw placement as compared to fluoroscopic-guided screws [24]. Given the varying results in the literature comparing robotic-assisted versus free-hand or fluoroscopically based pedicle screw placement, three recent high-quality meta-analyses have been performed based on published randomized controlled trials. Two of the meta-analyses demonstrated equivalent accuracy between the two techniques [25, 26], and a third demonstrated more superior accuracy with robotic assistance [27].

Studies comparing robotic-assisted pedicle screw placement versus 3D navigation techniques are fewer in number. Retrospective studies have demonstrated slightly higher accuracy with robotic-assisted screw placement compared to navigation-assisted screw placement. Laudato et al. demonstrated 79% versus 70% accuracy for robotic versus navigated screw placement, respectively [28]. Similarly, Roser et al. demonstrated 99% versus 92% accuracy for robotic versus navigated screw placement, respectively [29]. A recent meta-analysis demonstrated similar reduction in intraoperative and postoperative screw revision risk using robot or navigated screw placement, as compared to freehand techniques [30].

3.2 Proximal facet violation

The use of robotic-assisted pedicle screw placement can allow for precise preoperative or intraoperative planning of pedicle screw trajectories and accurate execution of the planned trajectory with assistance from the robotic arm. The ability to plan pedicle screw placement not only allows for optimization of the size and diameter of pedicle screws, but also allows for trajectories that avoid violation of the superior facet joint at the upper instrumented vertebral level. Violation of this joint can result in an increased risk of adjacent segment disease, which may compromise long-term clinical outcomes [31–33].

To date, three randomized-controlled trials [34–36] and one non-randomized prospective study [37] have demonstrated a reduced risk of superior facet joint violation when using robotic-assisted pedicle screw placement as compared to free-hand or fluoroscopically based techniques. Two meta-analyses also demonstrated similarly decreased violation of the superior facet joint when robotic assistance was utilized [27, 38].

3.3 Radiation

Radiation exposure is another area of concern for MISS surgeons, and significant exposure can occur when fluoroscopy is used in the absence of image guidance and navigation. Compared to freehand instrumentation techniques, most studies have demonstrated significantly decreased radiation exposure with robotic-assisted pedicle screw placement [18, 21, 29, 39]. Only two studies have demonstrated no significant difference in radiation exposure between the two instrumentation techniques [24, 28]. When broken down by source of radiation exposure, robotic assistance may result in higher doses to the patient [24], but lower doses to the surgeon [23]. Ultimately, inter-pretation of these studies is challenging because there can be significant variability in imaging acquisition protocols, surgeon experience, source of radiation detection, and specific freehand instrumentation techniques. Overall, however, the general body of evidence seems to support decreased radiation exposure with robot-assisted instru-mentation compared to traditional techniques that rely on fluoroscopy.

3.4 Operative time/efficiency

Several studies have attempted to compare the total operative time and time per screw insertion when using robot-assisted versus freehand techniques [18, 21, 29, 40]. However the comparative results of these studies can be confounded by variables related to approach (open versus percutaneous), the definition of operative time, and surgeon experience. Specific studies applicable to MISS have compared percutane-ous pedicle screw placement using a robot versus fluoroscopy-based techniques, but unfortunately they did not report operative time [41, 42]. A cadaveric study by Vaccaro et al. demonstrated that overall surgical time was similar between MISS pedicle screw placement using conventional fluoroscopy versus robot assistance [43]. The actual robot-assisted time per screw was actually lower, but this was offset by a longer setup time [43].

3.5 Impact on clinical outcomes and complications

Studies investigating the additive clinical benefit for robotic assistance in MISS compared to traditional fluoroscopically or 3D navigated MISS are lacking. Most of the literature compares traditional open procedures to robot-assisted MISS, and some of these studies have demonstrated decreased length of stay and faster postoperative recovery with the latter [44, 45]. Other studies comparing open procedures to MISS robot-assisted procedures have demonstrated lower infection rates and dural tear rates in the robot-assisted cohorts, but these studies were not powered to detect a significant difference [18, 23]. A recent study by Menger et al. projected robotic surgery to be more cost-effective secondary, in part, due to fewer revision surgeries and less postoperative complications [46]. As stated previously, none of these studies have specifically compared the additive benefit of robotic-assistance to traditional MISS procedures. If utilizing a robot allows surgeons who traditionally perform open surgery to convert to some MISS surgery with similar or improved instrumentation accuracy, decreased radiation, improved operative time, and potentially lower complications, the previously reported benefits of MISS surgery may become available to a greater number of patients.

4. Minimally invasive spine surgery robotic applications

4.1 Robotic-assisted transforaminal lumbar interbody fusion

Transforaminal lumbar interbody fusion (TLIF) allows for circumferential fusion, restoration of disc space height, and both direct and indirect neural decompression. Open TLIF has been associated with significant early postoperative morbidity secondary to extensive muscle retraction and dissection, which may result in increased postoperative pain, decreased mobility, and impaired overall function [47, 48]. In response to the limitations of open TLIF, the MI-TLIF was developed and has been shown to cause less postoperative pain, faster recovery, shorter hospitalization, and comparable functional outcomes to the open TLIF [49–51].

Traditionally, pedicle screws were placed percutaneously under fluoroscopic guidance for the MI-TLIF, resulting in potentially decreased accuracy and increased radiation exposure, as discussed in previous sections of this chapter. Until recently, the integration of spinal robotics into MI-TLIF has largely been confined to facilitating pedicle screw placement, and previous studies have reported on the feasibility and integration of robotics into the MI-TLIF workflow as well as the high pedicle screw placement accuracy [52–54]. Comparative studies assessing broader benefits of spine robot utilization versus traditional fluoroscopic or 3D navigation are lacking in the literature. De Biase et al., compared robot-assisted versus fluoroscopy-guided MI-TLIF procedures and reported no difference in operative time [55]. The study was limited by lack of comparative radiation, radiographic or functional outcomes between the two treatment groups [55].

A previous limitation of robotic MI-TLIF, as compared to 3D navigation, was that older robotic platforms did not allow for real-time navigation outside of pedicle screw placement. However, newer robotic software platforms now enable pre−/ intra-operative planning and navigation for tube placement, interbody cage placement, and disc space preparation (**Figure 1**). Evidence-based benefits of these real-time navigated features have yet to be established in the spinal literature. As robotic integration into MI-TLIF procedures continues to evolve and expand, further research is needed to investigate the possible additive benefit with regards to instrumentation accuracy, operative efficiency, radiation exposure, clinical outcomes, and fusion rates.

4.2 Robotic-assisted lateral and oblique lumbar interbody fusion

Lateral lumbar interbody fusion (LLIF) and oblique lumbar interbody fusion (OLIF) are minimally invasive techniques that can avoid some of the risks associated with anterior or posterior interbody approaches to the spinal column. Traditionally, after the interbody device is placed in LLIF and OLIF procedures in the lateral position, the patient is "flipped" to the prone position for pedicle screw instrumentation and posterior stabilization. Recent studies have begun to investigate the placement of posterior instrumentation in the lateral position, to avoid the "flip," and initial studies have demonstrated improved operative efficiency, less blood loss, and less postoperative ileus with single position lateral circumferential fusions [56].

One of the challenges of performing MISS posterior fixation in the lateral position is pedicle screw instrumentation. Interpreting fluoroscopic imaging, establishing accurate navigation, and the ergonomics of placing the down-sided pedicle screws can be difficult. Placement of robot-assisted pedicle screws in these procedures may offer a significant advantage as the robotic arm acts as a steady holding device, locking the trajectory of the planned pedicle screw, and thereby mitigating

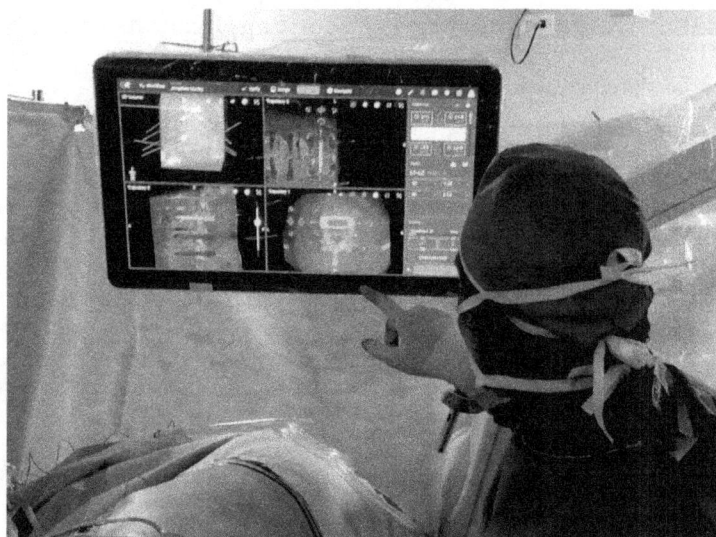

Figure 1.
Intraoperative planning using a spine robot's integrated navigation platform. This particular platform allows for intraoperative planning of pedicle screw trajectories, diameter, and length. Additionally, interbody placement can be planned, and navigated instruments can allow for targeted intraoperative disc preparation prior to interbody cage placement. Lastly, tube trajectories (if applicable) can also be planned.

some of the ergonomic challenges of placing these screws. The accuracy of pedicle screws with robot-assistance in the lateral position has been recently investigated and initial studies demonstrate 98% accuracy [57]. Images demonstrating this technique are shown in **Figure 2**.

As described in the MI-TLIF section, the latest iterations of software in some spinal robotics systems can allow for real-time navigation during tube placement, interbody cage placement, and disc space preparation. An additional benefit in the lateral or oblique position is that the robotic arm can be used to stabilize the retraction system, avoiding the need for a table mounted retractor (**Figure 3**). As these are all relatively recent advancements for robot-assisted LLIF and OLIF procedures, studies demonstrating a clinical benefit have yet to be performed.

4.3 Robotic-assisted MISS deformity correction

The majority of research on MISS has focused on addressing degenerative pathology, but as MISS continues to evolve, the utilization of MISS principals to address adult spinal deformity, without compromising outcomes, continues to be investigated. The traditional goals of adult spinal deformity surgery encompass restoration of sagittal and/or coronal balance, adequate neural element decompression, and achieving a solid arthrodesis. These goals may be achieved through MISS techniques – for example, lordosis can be restored through anterior column realignment procedures such as the LLIF and OLIF or posterior-based procedures such as MI-TLIF. Fixation can of course be achieved through percutaneous pedicle screw placement [58, 59]. In multi-level constructs, robotic assistance may have a cumulative benefit as the time saved at each subsequent level will have an additive benefit in longer deformity constructs. As discussed above, the use of a spinal robot may assist in executing these MISS procedures, just as is the case for patients with primarily degenerative pathology. However, evidence demonstrating the additive benefit of robotic-technology in MISS deformity procedures is sparse.

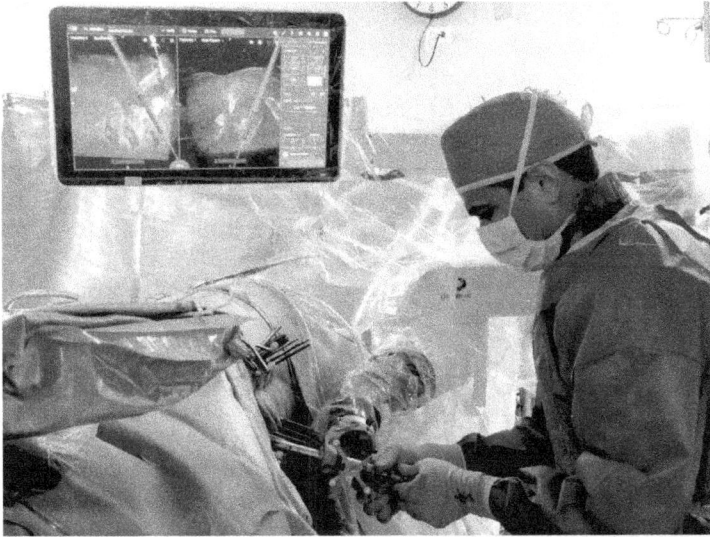

Figure 2.
Intraoperative placement of pre-planned pedicle screws for a multilevel lateral lumbar interbody fusion. In this image the down-sided pedicle screws are being placed based on the planned trajectory. The stabilized robotic arm facilitates the challenging placement of these screws, eliminates the need for interpretation of fluoroscopic imaging in the lateral position and improves the overall ergonomics and ease of placing these screws.

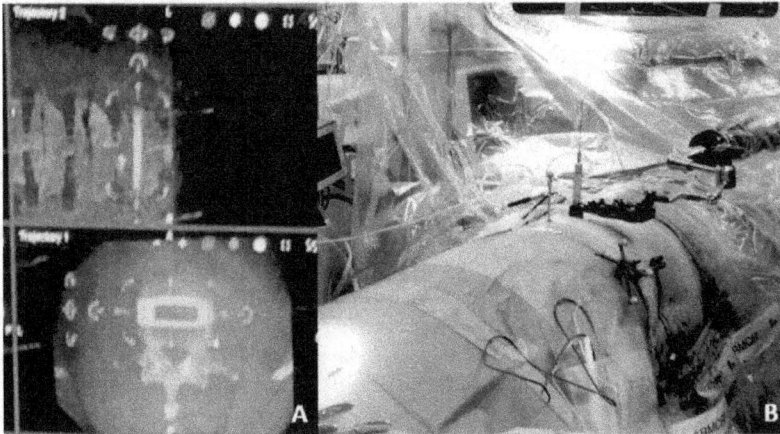

Figure 3.
The intraoperative navigation platform for this spine robot is used to plan the interbody placement in a multilevel lateral lumbar interbody fusion (A). The spine robot arm is then used to localize the trajectory of the planned retractor placement and the stabilized arm can be used to secure the retractor, avoiding the need for a table-mounted retractor (B).

One aspect of area robotic utilization within the field of adult spinal deformity that has received research interest is the safe and accurate placement of pelvic screw fixation. MISS percutaneous pelvic screw fixation using traditional fluoroscopy allows for less soft tissue dissection, as compared to the traditional open technique, which may result in a quicker recovery and less postoperative complications [60]. The additive use of robotic-assistance allows for preoperative planning, may increase accuracy, and decrease the technical difficulty in placing MISS pelvic fixation. A recent study demonstrated high accuracy with no intra- or postoperative complications using robotic-assistance for pelvic screw fixation in adult deformity patients [61].

5. Current limitations of robotic spine surgery

Over the past decade, robot-assisted surgery has played a significant role in the advancement of MISS, but there are limitations preventing its widespread adoption. These hurdles range from technical issues, cost, and operating room efficiency, to the learning curve associated with safely incorporating the robot into the operating room. Initial iterations of spine robots were met with concerns regarding instrument skiving and tool deflection, registration failures, and a lack of real-time navigation. Newer software iterations, as well as advancements in the robotic arm and its associated end-effectors have partly addressed these concerns. With regards to cost, there is no denying the significant capital expenditure required to obtain a spine robot; however, there may be a cost savings stemming from decreased postoperative complications secondary to improved instrumentation accuracy [46]. Further cost-effectiveness studies are needed, however, particularly with regards to MISS [62]. Lastly, there is a learning curve associated with performing safe robotic spinal surgery, but that learning curve may not be as high as previously conceived. One study demonstrated that 30 screws would need to be placed before a noticeable improvement in efficiency was observed [63], and two other studies demonstrated that between 13 and 20 cases may be needed to obtain proficiency in robotic screw placement [64, 65].

6. Future of robotic spine surgery

The safe implementation of robotic-assisted spine surgery in MISS continues to make progress and newer generations of spinal robots with improved software and real-time navigation will allow for the robot to be utilized for more than just pedicle screw instrumentation. Spine robots with real-time navigation currently allow for surgeons to plan tubular retractor trajectories, interbody placement, and navigated disc preparation. As the software continues to improve, magnetic resonance imaging (MRI)-based registration and navigation may allow for robot-assisted disc and ligamentum flavum resection as well as soft tissue tumor resection. Additionally, as burrs become compatible with the spinal robot, pre-operative planning and precise intra-operative execution of bony decompressions may become possible. Even in the domain of instrumentation, there is room for further advancement. While current spine robots only allow for assisted pedicle screw placement, future iterations may allow for fully automated pedicle screw placement. Yet another possibility is the syncing of intra-operative data from multiple robotic systems, which may one day enable machine learning and artificial intelligence algorithms to make real-time, intra-operative suggestions to surgeons based on previous surgeries. These future directions for robot-assisted MISS will likely continue to promote an increased integration and utilization of robotics into MISS.

Author details

Ram Kiran Alluri[1], Ahilan Sivaganesan[1], Avani S. Vaishnav[1]
and Sheeraz A. Qureshi[1,2]*

1 Hospital for Special Surgery, New York, NY, USA

2 Weill Cornell Medical College, New York, NY, USA

*Address all correspondence to: sheerazqureshimd@gmail.com

IntechOpen

References

[1] Shin DA, Kim KN, Shin HC, Yoon DH. The efficacy of microendoscopic discectomy in reducing iatrogenic muscle injury. J Neurosurg Spine. 2008;8:39-43.

[2] Ge DH, Stekas ND, Varlotta CG, et al. Comparative Analysis of Two Transforaminal Lumbar Interbody Fusion Techniques: Open TLIF Versus Wiltse MIS TLIF. Spine (Phila Pa 1976). 2019;44(9):E555–E560.

[3] Hockley A, Ge D, Vasquez-Montes D, et al. Minimally Invasive Versus Open Transforaminal Lumbar Interbody Fusion Surgery: An Analysis of Opioids, Nonopioid Analgesics, and Perioperative Characteristics. Glob Spine J. 2019;9(6):624-629.

[4] Kim CH, Easley K, Lee JS, et al. Comparison of Minimally Invasive Versus Open Transforaminal Interbody Lumbar Fusion. Glob Spine J. 2020;10 (2 Suppl):143S–150S.

[5] Mariscalco MW, Yamashita T, Steinmetz MP, Krishnaney AA, Lieberman IH, Mroz TE. Radiation exposure to the surgeon during open lumbar microdiscectomy and minimally invasive microdiscectomy: a prospective, controlled trial. Spine (Phila Pa 1976). 2011;36(3):255-260.

[6] Chou LB, Lerner LB, Harris AHS, Brandon AJ, Girod S, Butler LM. Cancer Prevalence among a Cross-sectional Survey of Female Orthopedic, Urology, and Plastic Surgeons in the United States. Womens Heal Issues. 2015;25(5):476-481.

[7] Lee WJ, Choi Y, Ko S, et al. Projected lifetime cancer risks from occupational radiation exposure among diagnostic medical radiation workers in South Korea. BMC Cancer. 2018;18(1):1206.

[8] Hamilton DK, Smith JS, Sansur CA, et al. Rates of new neurological deficit associated with spine surgery based on 108,419 procedures: a report of the scoliosis research society morbidity and mortality committee. Spine (Phila Pa 1976). 2011;36(15):1218-1228.

[9] Sukovich W, Brink-Danan S, Hardenbrook M. Miniature robotic guidance for pedicle screw placement in posterior spinal fusion: early clinical experience with the SpineAssist. Int J Med Robot. 2006;2:114-122.

[10] Y Barzilay, M Liebergall, A Fridlander, Knoller AF. Miniature robotic guidance for spine surgery-- introduction of a novel system and analysis of challenges encountered during the clinical development phase at two spine centres. Int J Med Robot. 2006;2(2):146-153.

[11] Kochanski RB, Lombardi JM, Laratta JL, Lehman RA, O'Toole JE. Image-Guided Navigation and Robotics in Spine Surgery. Neurosurgery. 2019;84(6):1179-1189.

[12] D'Souza M, Gendreau J, Feng A, Kim LH, Ho AL, Veeravagu A. Robotic-Assisted Spine Surgery: History, Efficacy, Cost, And Future Trends. Robot Surg. 2019;7(6):9-23.

[13] Kelly PJ. Neurosurgical robotics. Clin Neurosurg. 2002;49:136-158.

[14] Louw DF, Fielding T, McBeth PB, Gregoris D, Newhook P, Sutherland GR. Surgical robotics: a review and neurosurgical prototype development. Neurosurgery. 2004;54(3):525-537.

[15] Pechlivanis I, Kiriyanthan G, Engelhardt M, et al. Percutaneous placement of pedicle screws in the lumbar spine using a bone mounted miniature robotic system: first experiences and accuracy of screw placement. Spine (Phila Pa 1976). 2009;34:392-8.

[16] Tsai TH, Wu DS, Su YF, Wu CH, Lin CL. A retrospective study to validate an intraoperative robotic classification system for assessing the accuracy of kirschner wire (K-wire) placements with postoperative computed tomography classification system for assessing the accuracy of pedicle screw placements. Medicine (Baltimore). 2016;95:e4834.

[17] Kuo KL, Su YF, Wu CH, et al. Assessing the intraoperative accuracy of pedicle screw placement by using a bone-mounted miniature robot system through secondary registration. PLoS One. 2016;11:e0153235.

[18] Keric N, Doenitz C, Haj A, et al. Evaluation of robot-guided minimally invasive implantation of 2067 pedicle screws. Neurosurg Focus. 2017; 42:E11.

[19] van Dijk JD, van den Ende RPJ, Stramigioli S, Kochling M, Hoss N. Clinical pedicle screw accuracy and deviation from planning in robot-guided spine surgery: robot-guided pedicle screw accuracy. Spine (Phila Pa 1976). 2015;40:E986-991.

[20] Devito DP, Kaplan L, Dietl R, et al. Clinical acceptance and accuracy assessment of spinal implants guided with Spine Assist surgical robot: retrospective study. Spine (Phila Pa 1976). 2010;35:2109-15.

[21] Kantelhardt SR, Martinez R, Baerwinkel S, Burger R, Giese A, Rohde V. Perioperative course and accuracy of screw positioning in conventional, open robotic-guided and percutaneous robotic-guided, pedicle screw placement. Eur Spine J. 2011;20;860-868.

[22] Fan Y, Du J, Zhang J, et al. Comparison of accuracy of pedicle screw insertion among 4 guided technologies in spine surgery. Med Sci Monit. 2017;23:5960-5968.

[23] Le X, Tian W, Shi Z et al. Robot-assisted versus fluoroscopy assisted cortical bone trajectory screw instrumentation in lumbar spinal surgery: a matched-cohort comparison. World Neurosurg. 2018;120:e745–e751.

[24] Ringel F, Stuer C, Reinke A et al. Accuracy of robot-assisted placement of lumbar and sacral pedicle screws: a prospective randomized comparison to conventional freehand screw implantation. Spine (Phila Pa 1976). 2012;37(8):E496–E501.

[25] Gao S, Lv Z, Fang H. Robot-assisted and conventional freehand pedicle screw placement: a systematic review and meta-analysis of randomized controlled trials. Eur Spine J. 2018;27:920-930.

[26] Peng YN, Tsai LC, Hsu HC, Kao CH. Accuracy of robot-assisted versus conventional freehand pedicle screw placement in spine surgery: a systematic review and meta-analysis of randomized controlled trials. Ann Transl Med. 2020;8(13):824.

[27] Li HM, Zhang RJ, Shen CL. Accuracy of Pedicle Screw Placement and Clinical Outcomes of Robot-assisted Technique Versus Conventional Freehand Technique in Spine Surgery From Nine Randomized Controlled Trials: A Meta-analysis. Spine (Phila Pa 1976). 2020;45:E111–E119.

[28] Laudato PA, Pierzchala K, Schizas C. Pedicle Screw Insertion Accuracy Using O-Arm, Robotic Guidance, or Freehand Technique: A Comparative Study. Spine (Phila Pa 1976). 2018;43(6):E373–E378.

[29] Florian Roser 1, Marcos Tatagiba GM. Spinal robotics: current applications and future perspectives. Neurosurgery. 2013;72(Suppl 1):12-8.

[30] Staartjes VE, Klukowska AM, Schroder ML. Pedicle Screw Revision in

Robot-Guided, Navigated, and Freehand Thoracolumbar Instrumentation: A Systematic Review and Meta-Analysis. World Neurosurg. 2018;Aug(116):433-443.

[31] Bagheri SR, Alimohammadi E, Froushani AZ, Abdi A. Adjacent segment disease after posterior lumbar instrumentation surgery for degenerative disease: Incidence and risk factors. J Orthop Surg (Hong Kong). 2019;27:2309499019842378.

[32] Wang H, Ma L, Yang D et al. Incidence and risk factors of adjacent segment disease following posterior decompression and instrumented fusion for degenerative lumbar disorders. Medicine (Baltimore). 2017;96:E6032.

[33] Sakaura H, Miwa T, Yamashita T, Ohwada T. Cortical bone trajectory screw fixation versus traditional pedicle screw fixation for 2-level posterior lumbar interbody fusion: comparison of surgical outcomes for 2-level degenerative lumbar spondylolisthesis. J Neurosurg Spine. 2018;28:57-62.

[34] Hyun SJ, Kim KJ, Jahng TA, Kim HJ. Minimally invasive robotic versus open fluoroscopic-guided spinal instrumented fusions: a randomized controlled trial. Spine (Phila Pa 1976). 2017;42(6):353-358.

[35] Han X, Tian W, Liu Y et al. . Safety and accuracy of robot-assisted versus fluoroscopy-assisted pedicle screw insertion in thoracolumbar spinal surgery: a prospective randomized controlled trial. J Neurosurg Spine. 2019;1-8.

[36] Kim HJ, Jung WI, Chang BS, Lee CK, Kang KT, Yeom JS. A prospective, randomized, controlled trial of robot-assisted vs freehand pedicle screw fixation in spine surgery. Int J Med Robot. 2017;13(3).

[37] Zhang Q, Xu YF, Tian W. Comparison of Superior-Level Facet Joint Violations Between Robot-Assisted Percutaneous Pedicle Screw Placement and Conventional Open Fluoroscopic-Guided Pedicle Screw Placement. Orthop Surg. 2019;11(5):850-856.

[38] Zhou LP, Zhang RJ, Li HM, Shen CL. omparison of Cranial Facet Joint Violation Rate and Four Other Clinical Indexes Between Robot-assisted and Freehand Pedicle Screw Placement in Spine Surgery: A Meta-analysis. Spine (Phila Pa 1976). 2020;45(22):E1532-40.

[39] Lieberman IH, Hardenbrook MA, Wang JC, Guyer RD. Assessment of pedicle screw placement accuracy, procedure time, and radiation exposure using a miniature robotic guidance system. J Spinal Disord Tech. 2012;25(5):241-248.

[40] Solomiichuk V, Fleischhammer J, Molligaj G et al. Robotic versus fluoroscopy-guided pedicle screw insertion for metastatic spinal disease: a matched-cohort comparison. Neurosurg Focus. 2017;42(5):E13.

[41] Yang JS, He B, Tian F, et al. Accuracy of Robot-Assisted Percutaneous Pedicle Screw Placement for Treatment of Lumbar Spondylolisthesis: A Comparative Cohort Study. Med Sci Monit. 2019;25: (2479-2487).

[42] Fayed I, Tai A, Triano M, et al. Robot-Assisted Percutaneous Pedicle Screw Placement: Evaluation of Accuracy of the First 100 Screws and Comparison with Cohort of Fluoroscopy-guided Screws. World Neurosurg. 2020;143:e492–e502.

[43] Vaccaro AR, Harris JA, Hussain MM, et al. Assessment of Surgical Procedural Time, Pedicle Screw Accuracy, and Clinician Radiation Exposure of a Novel Robotic Navigation System Compared With Conventional Open and Percutaneous Freehand

Techniques: A Cadaveric Investigation. Glob Spine J. 2020;10(7):814-825.

[44] Hyun SJ, Kim KJ, Jahng TA, Kim HJ. Minimally invasive robotic versus open fluoroscopic-guided spinal instrumented fusions. Spine (Phila Pa 1976). 2017;42:353-358.

[45] Lucio JC, Vanconia RB, Deluzio KJ, Lehmen JA, Rodgers JA, Rodgers WB. Economics of less invasive spinal surgery: an analysis of hospital cost differences between open and minimally invasive instrumented spinal fusion procedures during the perioperative period. Risk Manag Heal Policy. 2012;5:65-74.

[46] Menger RP, Savardekar AR, Farokhi F, Sin A. A cost-effectiveness analysis of the integration of robotic spine technology in spine surgery. Neurospine. 2018;15(3):216-224.

[47] Styf JR, Willen J. The effects of external compression by three different retractors on pressure in the erector spine muscles during and after posterior lumbar spine surgery in humans. Spine (Phila Pa 1976). 1998;23(3):354-358.

[48] Gejo R, Matsui H, Kawaguchi Y, Tsuji H. Serial changes in trunk muscle performance after posterior lumbar surgery. Spine (Phila Pa 1976). 1999;24:1023-8.

[49] Peng CWB, Yue WM, Poh SY, Yeo W, Tan SB. Clinical and radiological outcomes of minimally invasive versus open transforaminal lumbar interbody fusio. Spine (Phila Pa 1976). 2009;34(13):1385-1389.

[50] Seng C, Siddiqui MA, Wong KPL, Zhang K, Yeo W, Tan SB, Yue WM. Five-year outcomes of minimally invasive versus open transforaminal lumbar interbody fusion: a matched-pair comparison study. Spine (Phila Pa 1976). 2013;38(23):2049-2055.

[51] Lee KH, Yue WM, Yeo W, Soeharno H, Tan SB. Clinical and radiological outcomes of open versus minimally invasive transforaminal lumbar interbody fusion. Eur Spine J. 2012;21:2265-2270.

[52] Du JP, Fan Y, Liu JJ, Zhang JN, Liu SC, Hao D. Application of Gelatin Sponge Impregnated with a Mixture of 3 Drugs to Intraoperative Nerve Root Block Combined with Robot-Assisted Minimally Invasive Transforaminal Lumbar Interbody Fusion Surgery in the Treatment of Adult Degenerative Scoliosis: A Clinical Observation Inclduing 96 Patients. World Neurosurg. 2017;108:791-797.

[53] Chenin L, Peltier J, Lefranc M. Minimally invasive transforaminal lumbar interbody fusion with the ROSA(TM) Spine robot and intraoperative flat-panel CT guidance. Acta Neurochir. 2016;158:1125-1128.

[54] Snyder LA. Integrating robotics into a minimally invasive transforaminal interbody fusion workflow. Neurosurg Focus. 2018;45:V4.

[55] De Biase G, Gassie K, Garcia D, et al. Perioperative Comparison of Robotic-Assisted versus Fluoroscopy-Guided Minimally Invasive Transforaminal Lumbar Interbody Fusion (TLIF). World Neurosurg. 2021;Feb 4:S1878-8750.

[56] Buckland AJ, Ashayeri K, Leon C, et al. Single position circumferential fusion improves operative efficiency, reduces complications and length of stay compared with traditional circumferential fusion. Spine J. 13:S1529-9430(20)31217-1.

[57] Huntsman KT, Riggleman JR, Ahrendtsen LA, Ledonio CG. Navigated robot-guided pedicle screws placed successfully in single-position lateral lumbar interbody fusion. J Robot Surg. 2020;14(4):643-647.

[58] Berjano P, Cecchinato R, Sinigaglia A. Anterior column realignment from a lateral approach for the treatment of severe sagittal imbalance: a retrospective radiographic study. Eur Spine J. 2015;24 (Suppl 3):433-438.

[59] Leveque JC, Yanamadala V, Buchlak Q, Sethi RK. Correction of severe spinopelvic mismatch: decreased blood loss with lateral hyperlordotic interbody grafts as compared with pedicle subtraction osteotomy. Neurosurg Focus. 2917;43:E15.

[60] Tanaka M, Fujiwara Y, Uotani K, Maste P, Yamauchi T. C-Arm-Free Circumferential Minimally Invasive Surgery for Adult Spinal Deformity: Technical Note. World Neurosurg. 2020;143:235-246.

[61] Hyun SJ, Kim KJ, Jahng TA. S2 alar iliac screw placement under robotic guidance for adult spinal deformity patients: technical note. Eur Spine J. 2017;26(8):2198-2203.

[62] Fiani B, Quadri SA, Farooqui M, et al. Impact of robot-assisted spine surgery on health care quality and neurosurgical economics: A systemic review. Neurosurg Rev. 2020;43(1):17-25.

[63] Siddiqui MI, Wallace DJ, Salazar LM, Vardiman AB. RobotAssisted Pedicle Screw Placement: Learning Curve Experience. World Neurosurg. 2019;130:e417–e422.

[64] Schatlo B, Martinez R, Alaid A et al. Unskilled unawareness and the learning curve in robotic spine surgery. Acta Neurochir. 2015;157:1819-1823.

[65] Hu X, Lieberman IH. What is the learning curve for robotic-assisted pedicle screw placement in spine surgery? Clin Orthop Relat Res. 2014;472:1839-1844.